The 'Be Rad' Bedroom Body Book
By Bradley of B-Rad TV

© 2018 The Creative Divide: Bradley of B-Rad TV
First Published on Kindle in 2016
The 'Be Rad' Bedroom Body Book, its contents, cover and images, are the property of the Author, Bradley of B-Rad TV

Table of Contents

1. HOW MY JOURNEY BEGAN..**PAGE 1**

2. WHY SHOULD YOU EXERCISE?...**PAGE 7**

3. WILL THIS WORK FOR ME?..**PAGE 11**

4. **UNDERSTANDING YOUR BODY:** BUILDING MUSCLE AND LOSING FAT - BLOOD - BREATHING..................................**PAGE 15**

5. **NUTRITION:** FOOD GROUPS - EATING TO LOSE WEIGHT - EATING AROUND TRAINING...**PAGE 21**

6. **THE 'BE RAD' NUTRITION PLAN:** FOOD PREPARATION GUIDE - MEAL PLANS - WHAT TIME SHOULD I EAT? - HEALTHY TREATS - GETTING INTO A ROUTINE..**PAGE 29**

7. **MUSCLES OF THE BODY**..**PAGE 43**

8. **WEIGHT TRAINING EQUIPMENT**..**PAGE 53**

9. **WEIGHT TRAINING: WHAT YOU NEED TO KNOW:** WHEN SHOULD I TRAIN? - REPETITIONS AND SETS - SUPER SETS - PYRAMID SETS - TARGETING MUSCLE GROUPS - REST & CORRECT FORM........**PAGE 57**

10. **THE 'BE RAD' BEDROOM WORKOUT PLAN:** WORKOUT STRUCTURE - THE WORKOUT PLANS...**PAGE 65**

11. **THE EXERCISES:** HOW I KEEP MY LEGS STRONG - STRETCHING AND FLEXING - CORE - DAY ONE: CHEST AND ARMS - DAY TWO: BACK AND ARMS - DAY THREE: SHOULDERS AND ARMS.........**PAGE 71**

12. **WHAT HAS THIS 3-MONTH JOURNEY BEEN LIKE FOR ME?**
.......**PAGE 145**

1. HOW MY JOURNEY BEGAN

Hi guys, Bradley from B-Rad TV here (*www.youtube.com/bradtelevision*), speaking to you for the first time in written form, which hopefully won't stop any of my energy or enthusiasm for life from bursting through! Firstly, let me just say I'm not a professionally qualified personal trainer or nutritionist, I'm just a guy, a guy who has been exercising and dieting in a number of ways for the past decade and experienced a variety of results, and now, I am presenting my knowledge to you.

When I first starting working out I starved myself; I would skip breakfast, run to college, have a milkshake for lunch, run to the gym, workout, have a protein shake, run home, then have a tuna wrap. This was an eating disorder and an obsession with exercise caused by body dysmorphia. I was malnourished and regularly got colds, and this was when I was 17-19, I seriously believe I stunted my growth and affected my body for life by living like this during years I was still developing.

In my early twenties I went the other way, I believed I was small and worthless, so started lifting heavy, *heavy* weights and eating 5000+ calories a day. I would be in the gym 2 hours everyday 6 days a week. Following the bodybuilding workouts was healthy enough, but following their diets was not. Little did I realise the diets I was following were intended for giants on steroids, their insane metabolisms and enlarged stomachs could process the huge quantities of food they put into their bodies on a daily basis, whereas mine could not. I would eat a high-calorie meal replacement bar, then have a pre-workout shake, then workout for 2 hours, then have a custom-made shake of ice cream, walnuts, milk, banana and protein powder (which was close to 2000 calories itself), then two tins of tuna with a plate *full* of pasta, a few hours later I'd eat a 6 egg omelette on five bits of toast, then a few hours after that I'd have 2 chicken breasts with another plate of pasta and then before bed a double serving of protein powder with milk. The bulk on my shoulders, chest and arms meant I didn't *look* fat, but I was unhealthily overweight and was actually carrying around *a lot* of excess fat, both externally and internally. I could feel the pressure on my heart and insides; I was bloated all the time, had problems breathing, sleeping and going to the toilet, I spent all my money on food, supplements and gym memberships, I damaged my joints and ached when I had to walk anywhere, I had nose bleeds constantly (to the point where I would wake up in the morning with my face and pillows covered with blood). During this time I was the physically biggest and strongest I have ever been, and probably ever will be, but I was sluggish, slow, seriously unhealthy and eating my way to an early grave.

Then as it does, life took its toll and after a series of losses I became severely depressed; I spent a couple of years at the bottom of a bottle scraping through life. Without my friends and family I would have been homeless or dead. During this time I didn't go to the gym and if I did find the strength to eat (or wasn't too sick from drinking) it definitely wouldn't have been anything with any nutritional value, I lost about four stone in a matter of months. Worryingly though, I remember noticing that my breathing became more regular, smoother and easier; which just goes to show how unhealthy I must have been when I was obsessed with getting as big as I possibly could.

Slowly, with lots of support from my friends and family, I managed to take control of my life again. I looked at every part of my life: what I wanted for myself, how I wanted to live, who I wanted to be and of course my physical condition. I managed to say no to the alcohol and eventually started eating regularly again. I couldn't afford a regular gym membership (that's how bad things had got at this point) but I did get a set of small dumbbells for my room, and I went to work on making myself *healthy*. It was in this time of self-discovery I first began meditating and *really* looking deep within myself. Over time I began to discover fragments of peace and contentment I didn't know existed. Appearance was no longer a concern of mine, after being as low as I had, my guilt, shame and ego had been shattered. It really wasn't important what other people thought of me as I tried to put my life back on track, I had to do it for *me*. For the first time the motivation to life weights and regulate my diet was primarily for health reasons. That said, the boost to my confidence and the improvement in my wellbeing I noticed when I began exercising again was incredible. It gave me a routine, something to focus and work on, something to feel like I'd achieved during a time I felt utterly pathetic; lifting weights and preparing my own meals played a *massive* part in me saving my own life.

From here I began eating mostly natural food; fruits, vegetables, wholegrain breads, pastas and rice, lean meats, nuts, seeds and milk. In regular portion sizes three times a day; breakfast, lunch and dinner, with healthy snacks in between if I needed an energy boost. I became a lot more adaptable with when I ate as well; in the past I'd been overwhelmed and stressed about fitting my healthy eating around a normal life as I tried desperately to stick to whatever routine I was copying, but as I started my new, busier life in Central London I found living and thinking fluidly helped me live in balance during what was a very unbalanced, unpredictable time. A large part of this was due to my new, open, accepting and abundant mindset; I'm of the opinion that the *mind* is the most powerful tool in sculpting the body and life you want.

After a while following my personal bedroom workout routines and preparing my own healthy meals my body started functioning better that I could ever remember it functioning; I could breathe deeply, my joints didn't ache and I would sleep right through the night. Living in balance brought me to a healthy bodyweight, my hair was thick, my skin was flawless and my head was clear. I had been dragged through the dirt by life and been lower than I ever thought it was possible to be, but I had emerged victorious, enthused and happy to be alive. It's an incredible feeling and I want as many of you as possible to feel that way as well.

Finally, after much trial and error, I'm in a place where I completely understand my own body; I know what and when to eat and exactly how to train to ensure my mind and body are operating at their full potential. Not only this, but I'm also able to physically sculpt myself into any form I desire; if I want to broaden my shoulders or fill the sleeves of my t-shirts or even lose size healthily to look leaner and less bulky, I know the most efficient way to do so. I feel like I've developed some sort of super power! When the reality of it is that I read, listened, watched, learned, practiced, tried, failed, succeeded, failed, tried, gave up, struggled, tried again, read even more, listened, practiced and trained, trained, trained. If you are willing to put in the *hard work*, and lots of it, you can transform your mind, body and life as well!

Currently, I'm the busiest I've ever been and I'm travelling around the world with work; I've managed to turn my life into an *adventure* I want to have. Though always having ups and downs, which is what life will always be, I'm glad when I wake up in the mornings and I'm so thankful for another day on this planet.

I try to live in balance but also want to experience and live the fullest life possible, which means sometimes I end up going a bit too far, *really* too far sometimes, then shrugging my shoulders and saying, "Oh well, life is for living." But I paid the price for this carefree thinking after living to excess and burning out, both physically and mentally, during the last few months of 2015. I was waking up too hungover from alcohol to eat the cold junk food in my fridge. My sleep became disturbed and I was drinking most nights, alone, until the Sun was rising. I stopped answering my phone and didn't want to leave my room because I'd become so ashamed of myself. That was not how I wanted to start the New Year; I knew I was so much better than that and I decided it was time to sort myself out. So I set myself the goal that for 3 months, from 1st January 2016 – 31st March 2016, I was going to put *all* of my knowledge into practice and live as healthily as I knew how. Contained within these pages is a simple to understand guide on exactly how I ate, trained and lived during those 3 months. You can see the results in the images below...

Beginning of January 2016

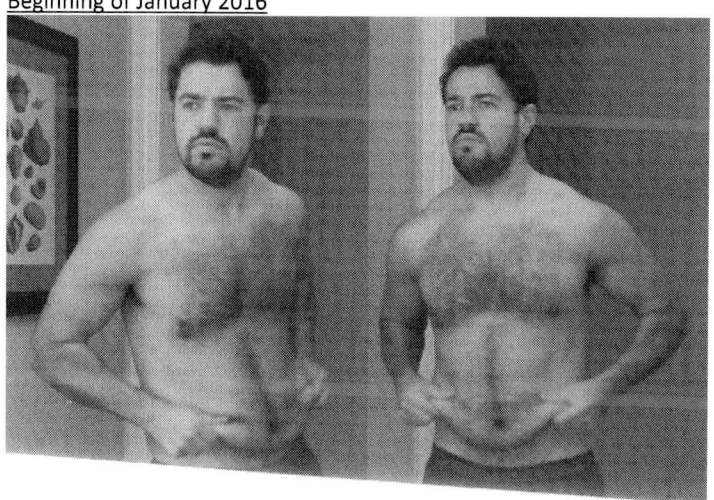

End of March 2016

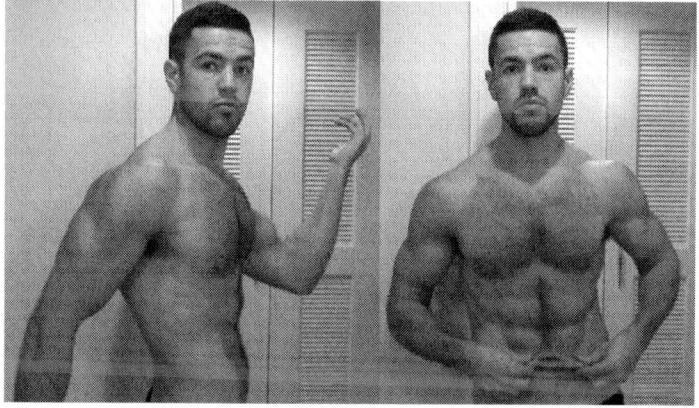

I hope I inspire and encourage you, but most of all, I want to awaken the strength within *YOU!* You might need the push from someone else to find your power, just as I did, but I promise that within you there is a source of strength and hope that you can use to build the life you want and deserve! Let's do this guys! Let's BE RAD!

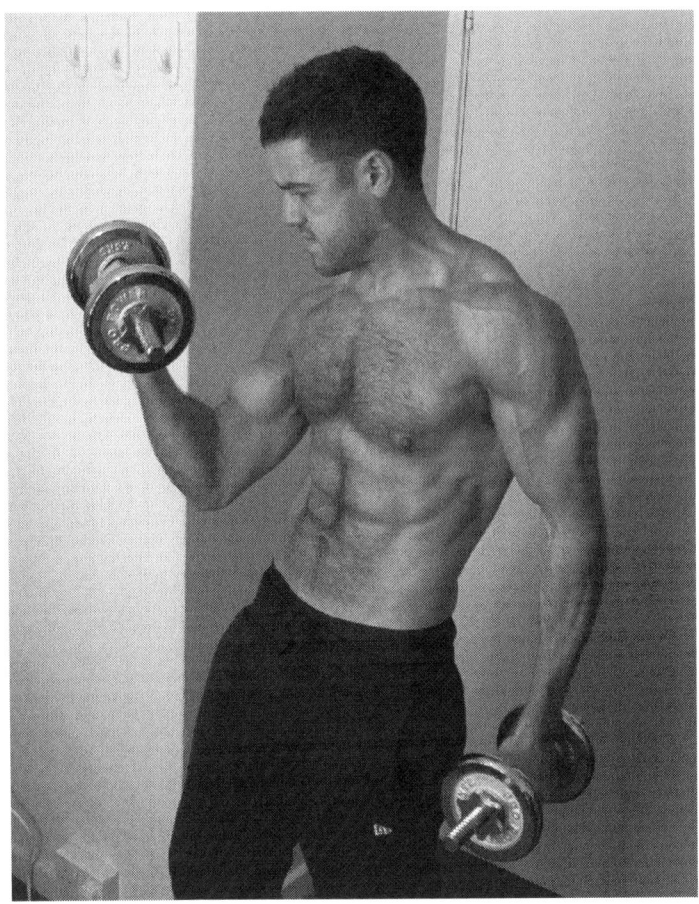

2. WHY SHOULD YOU EXERCISE?

There is only one person on the planet that can tell you that you are overweight, and that is YOU! If you weigh 21 stone and only eat burgers but are genuinely happy with yourself and your life, then good for you. If you truly love and respect yourself and are living the happiest, fullest life you think you possibly can, then brilliant! There are millions of people half your size that can't say the same thing. For my part though, I know when I stop exercising for a while, or start drinking too many energy drinks or eating too much fast food, I sweat more, I get out of breath quicker, my energy levels are unpredictable, I get tired and irritable and then because of all of this my overall mood sinks dramatically which sends me further down the spiral of decline. I'm so in touch with my own body now I can tell straight away when I'm beginning to become 'overweight' *in my opinion*. To me, overweight means:

HAVING AN EXCESS AMOUNT OF BODYWEIGHT THAT AFFECTS THE DAILY FUNCTIONING OF MY BODY

It's not about what you like *at all*, it's how you feel, move and function. If you get out of breath walking up the stairs to your seat in the cinema, wheezing and sweating as you navigate your large popcorn around your 48inch waist and find that a relaxing experience then you're not overweight as far as I'm concerned; if you are at peace with yourself and satisfied with your life then you have nothing to worry about. The only obvious negatives would be the medical facts about the pressure on your heart and the risk of diseases that might lead to an early death, but if you have accepted that and are perfectly at peace, I must say I envy you. Personally though, I can only imagine that struggling for breath, sweating profusely, having limited mobility and having a higher risk of DEATH would cause me a great deal of mental and physical anguish.

I know if I suddenly saw a member of my family had put on a dangerous amount of weight I would address the issue because I don't want anyone I care about to be in pain. If they turned round and told me they were at peace, it would be very hard for me to accept. How could they have accepted such pain and negative health implications for themselves? I would let them live their life how they intended, but without being a nagging pest I would never be afraid to let them know how worried I was about them. I'm mentioning this because I want to reassure you that if your loved ones are worried about your weight, it's because they're worried about *you*. Of course if you have idiots or bullies in your life that call you names and throw around the word 'fat', their opinions should be of no concern to you, their words only have the power you give them. There is only *one* person you can call you overweight, remember? And that is *you*.

If you decide that you do consider yourself overweight and have committed to changing your life (if you are reading this I assume you have) then I must say **WELL DONE**! Admitting mistakes and problems to ourselves is one of the hardest things we ever have to do in this world. I'm not going to lie, it's going to be a long, tough journey; it's going to involve gruelling hard work that will make you sweat, cry and ache...at first. But then you will start to breathe easier, sweat less, walk quicker, be able to carry more, pick things off the floor easier and generally move much more smoothly and without discomfort. Before long you'll feel so empowered and confident you'll walk with your head held high and you'll be glowing with self-respect and clarity of purpose. People will begin to notice, and often those who lose weight think the comments they receive are solely because of the weight loss, but what I think people are *really* commenting on is the newfound confidence and power that seems to radiate from those taking control of their own lives. It's the hour after hour of training they see when they look you in the eyes, the dedication, self-control and self-knowledge of your life and where you are going.

This confidence and control will *always* improve the quality of your life. When you walk into a job interview and your clothes fit well, you stride with confidence and you have the alert look of someone in control of their life, how do you think that looks to a potential employer? It looks incredible. If you have your mind, body and life in order you should make short work of any tasks they set out for you. When you go to social gatherings and so many negative people moan about their lives but do nothing about it the atmosphere can be really draining, what do you think happens when you, a beacon of dedication and hard work walks in? Some people might get jealous, some might get afraid and some will stand there in awe. I'm not trying to use this as some kind of ego-boosting motivation, but I do want to let you know that if you take control of your own life, mind and body, you will find it easier to survive and progress in what is still, sadly, a dog-eat-dog world.

Commit to your journey and see it through. You will feel better than you have ever felt, look better than you've ever looked and live a longer, happier life.

You are going to change *your* life and you're never going to regret it...

3. WILL THIS WORK FOR ME?

This book, and all the information in it, is for anyone and everyone. Exercising regularly and eating a healthy, balanced diet will benefit you no matter who you are or where you are on your journey of life. You will never be as young as you are right now, so make a start! Of course you know your own body and should take your injuries and abilities into consideration, but never let them deter you from doing what needs to be done.

Injuries can strike us down when we least expect it and how we deal with the aftermath of accidents will determine the course of the rest of our lives. After a major sporting injury I couldn't walk for almost a year and was in and out of hospital numerous times. I've had a total of 8 operations on one of my knees, I almost lost my leg from the knee down and the joint was irreparably damaged; they said I was too young for a complete knee replacement but I've been promised one for when I'm older, hooray... This whole experience was very shocking and life altering, but I picked myself up, dusted myself off and adapted. I worked out with a small set of dumbbells lying on my mattress and punched the air thousands of times to get my heart going. My body didn't look muscly or athletic, but I felt healthy and kept my organs functioning well at a time I could have let my mind and body stagnate. I'd had fractured pieces of bone removed, warped muscles tightened back to position, cells cloned and reattached, then shaved down, I was in a wheelchair, in a splint, had stitches, staples, bandages, crutches, morphine and other flavours of pain killers, anti-inflammatories, hydrotherapy, the list goes on, but I committed to my physiotherapy and learned to walk again. Now, years later, if you saw me walking down the street you'd never know it had happened. I adapted lots of the exercises featured later in this book around my temporary immobility, and so long as you understand your body and any ailments affecting it, you can do the same.

That injury has affected me for life. I have never been able to do weighted exercises on my legs or perform any large full-body, compound exercises that would put my knee at risk (squats, deadlifts, etc.). I have had to train very smart to avoid injuring myself further. My knee is a very high-risk joint for me but I have found ways to strengthen it so that it doesn't affect my day-to-day activities, which I will detail later. Also, all of the exercise I do, (so all of the exercises contained in this book) take my injury into consideration. I couldn't make such a broad statement now as "If you have a knee injury or damaged joints all of these exercises are perfect for you" because every injury is different and I would never want to mislead anyone. Only *you* can know what you are physically capable of, but the reality is that I have one much weaker leg and a severely damaged joint but I perform all of these exercises regularly and benefit greatly from it.

Sometimes I hear people say they are nervous or embarrassed about joining a gym; if this is you don't worry, it's very common and was even me when I first started training. In recent years it has become even more of a problem for people though, due to this deeply unpleasant, elitist, almost bullying culture that has developed online that mocks gym goers who don't workout correctly or wear the 'proper' clothes or fit nicely into their image of a perfect gym. These people are of *no concern* to you because *you* are only concerned with *you*, while they are worrying about their social standing or bringing people down, *you* are working, thinking, committed and driven. You have no time or mental capacity to spare for these negative people because *you* are completely dedicated to improving yourself. THERE IS NOTHING ELSE. If you need help adopting this mindset or just a confidence boost before joining a gym this book will be of great help to you. It details the incredibly effective workouts I used to transform myself in my tiny, single bedroom over the course of a 3-month period. I promise you, the mental evolution you experience after completing a journey of self-improvement like this is just as great, if not greater, than the physical evolution; and you will be more than ready to join any gym you want.

Say you've never even exercised before, let alone been to a gym. Don't worry, I'll say it again, YOU WILL NEVER BE AS YOUNG AS YOU ARE RIGHT NOW. The past is done, but by working on yourself in the present you greatly increase the potential of your future. Don't dwell on the past if you do feel as though you've been neglecting yourself, you have decided to make a change and that is far more important.

You may have noticed from things I've said already, or if you've skipped ahead through this book, that most of my workouts involve lifting weights. When I speak to people this seems to be a huge mental roadblock when it comes to how they view exercise, especially with women. Whenever I recommend lifting weights as a way to improve the quality of your health and wellbeing the most popular response I get from ladies is, "I don't want to get big and muscly." Don't worry, unless you set yourself that target and seriously look into what it takes to transform yourself that much it won't happen. The routines and diets in this book will make you lose excess fat, strengthen and tone you, but will not turn you into a behemoth. The reasons I swear by weightlifting as a form of exercise will become apparent as you read on.

This book is ideally suited to anyone on a budget, we will only be using 4 pieces of equipment: a set of dumbbells, an inflatable Swiss ball, an exercise mat and a set of press-up handles (which collectively can cost the same amount as one month's gym membership if you shop around). Also, when I started planning and preparing all of my own meals I stopped eating out as much, stopped impulse buying food that I didn't really need and didn't have any excess food going to waste. I saved *a lot* of money living in a routine like this, even only for 3 months.

This book is also for busy people; you will be saving a lot of time by not needing to pack a gym bag, travel to a gym or wait for someone to stop using a piece of equipment. The workouts can be done at any time of day and even shortened or adapted to fit around your schedule. The meals I prepare take a matter of minutes and create a *very* small amount of washing up.

The exercises can also be performed in a *very* limited amount of space, (so you won't need to wait for your family to vacate the living room to do them). Personally, I performed all of these exercises in a room smaller than the average prison cell; I had to fit my legs between a cupboard and hanging rail of clothes to perform press-ups and any other full-body length exercises, I had to do all of my vertical pressing exercises stood in exactly the same place to avoid smashing the light that hangs from my ceiling, for any sweeping shoulder exercises I had to lift the weight over the bed being careful to avoid all of my belongings on the bed which I'd had to move off the floor area to exercise in the first place! So when I say you can perform all of these workouts in your bedroom, I *really* mean it.

The efficiency and simplicity of the exercises and meals means you don't need to be an accomplished athlete or chef to master them. Anyone can, and I'm sure *you* will. The exercises are also completely adaptable to your strength and fitness levels, so they are equally as effective if you've never lifted a weight before or if you're a seasoned gym-goer looking for a new routine to break through a training plateau.

This is a battle you have decided to fight, a fight for the life you want! Your only opponent is yourself. When you wake up on a cold morning or get home late from work, the only person who will stop you from exercising or preparing a healthy meal is *you*. When you look in the mirror, what sort of person do *you* want to see staring back at you? I want you to see someone who decided what they wanted and worked for it, however hard or impossible it seemed and no matter the cost. If you put in the work, you *WILL* get the results. Life is really that simple.

NOW LET'S GET STARTED...

4. UNDERSTANDING YOUR BODY

Before you begin exercising it is very important you understand how your body works, so you can understand why you should exercise and eat a certain way. Understanding your body means you can be more adaptable with the workouts and meals because you will *know* the reasoning behind what you are doing and the results it will get you.

Your body is a biological machine; bones and joints pulled to and fro by muscles, a heart pumping blood through your arteries, lungs that fill with air and expel the harmful chemicals, a digestive system constantly processing our food into nutrients and waste, kidneys and liver filtering urine and blood, and a brain sending electrical signals everywhere without us even realising it. When all of these processes are functioning correctly you feel good, when they under unnecessary strain and not functioning correctly, you feel bad. It's simple. Like any machine, if you treat it well, it will work better for longer, if you treat it poorly it will perform poorly and break prematurely. But unlike other 'machines' there are *no* replacements, *no* spares and *no* part exchanges; we get one physical self and I urge you to take care of it.

Building Muscle and Losing Fat

The excess fat on your body is stored energy, you need to create a demand for this stored energy in order to lose the fat; this demand is created by exercising. If at the same time you eat a regulated and nutritious diet, making sure you are not eating an excess amount of food, you won't put the fat straight back on.

If your body is a machine, then the muscles are the moving parts and the food we eat is the fuel. Our muscles are what use the energy from our food and fat stores. So essentially your muscles eat away at your fat as you exercise. The larger your muscles, the more fuel they require to work, whether that comes from food or fat stores. Therefore, **THE BIGGER YOUR MUSCLES THE MORE FAT THEY WILL BURN AWAY.** This is science fact; whether you are a man, woman, old or young, the more muscle you have, the easier and quicker it will be to lose your excess body fat.

So, your NUMBER ONE priority for losing weight should be to increase the size and strength of your muscles; to work on your body and turn it into a machine that *demands* more fuel. The most efficient way of building bigger, stronger, more fuel-hungry muscles is by lifting weights.

As well as your muscles consuming fuel (from food or fat stores) when you exert yourself with lifting weights, they also continue to use fuel for many hours afterwards as well. When you lift weights you make small tears in your muscles, which are repaired by your incredible body, and repaired very slightly larger; this is why your muscles grow. To facilitate this repairing process, which takes time, your body requires good quality food. Long after your weightlifting workout, your body is still consuming that fuel and using it to repair your muscles. You'll be burning the fat stores away while you brush your teeth, do the washing up and even while you sleep!

Spending hours and hours pounding away on a cross-trainer or a treadmill is *not* the most efficient way to lose weight and keep it off. Of course, you will lose weight and cardiovascular exercise is incredibly good for you, but if you want the most effective and long-lasting fat-loss solution then start lifting weights.

I haven't been on a treadmill, bike or cross trainer in years. The only cardio exercise I do is slow-paced swimming and very low weights with lots of repetitions. Due to my aforementioned knee injury I simply can't do any traditional cardio so I've had to rely on lifting weights and dieting, in doing so I've turned my body into a furnace that burns fuel all day and all night.

When you lose fat, you lose it all over your body at the same time; there is no such thing as 'spot reduction'. You can't say, "I only want to lose my belly", our body just doesn't work like that. Genetically we are all different and some people store more fat on their mid-rift, some on their thighs and some on their neck and face. The only way to reduce the excess fat in these places is to focus on strengthening and working out your *entire* body.

Any movement you make involves your muscles using energy, that's ANY movement; walking, clapping your hands, cleaning the house, carrying the shopping, picking an object off the floor, ANYTHING. If you live a sedentary lifestyle, start taking the stairs instead of the lift or walking twenty minutes to the shops rather than driving. Simple things like this will gradually start to increase your strength, stamina and overall fitness levels.

In an old job I had a co-worker who kept saying she wanted to get fit, but there were no gyms near where she lived, she couldn't afford a cross-trainer, she had an endless list of excuses. I explained she didn't need a gym to exercise, which confused her for some reason, so I thought I'd demonstrate my point, or rather get her to demonstrate it for me. That day we'd had a box of leaflets delivered to the shop, a large stack of leaflets in a small cardboard box that while it wasn't dangerously heavy, it still had a noticeable amount of weight to it. I told her to pick the box up, bending at the knees and keeping her back straight, which she did. I then told her to carry the box to the other side of the room, only about 5m to walk, and put the box down in the same manner, which she did. "That's not exercise," she smirked. I then told her to do it 1000 times. She laughed, but then did it again, and again, and again, with me counting the amount she was doing. She almost made it to twenty reps before giving up, out of breath and red in the face. Every muscle in her body was suddenly activated and working hard to lift and carry that box, and her heart was pumping much, much faster. This was exercise, ANY movement can be an exercise and ANYTHING can be used to exercise with (so long as it is safe to do so), there is nothing stopping you from working your muscles and getting your heart pumping.

Blood

Every process in your body relies on blood travelling around your body through veins and arteries; it carries oxygen, nutrients and white blood cells to fight infections (amongst other things). When you exercise your muscles get filled with blood which gives them all the fuel they need to function. Stretching before, after and even during a workout ensures that your muscles are awake and there is a healthy amount of blood flowing to all the parts of your body that are about to need it. This is why 'warming-up', however slight, is always necessary because it prepares your body for the exertion that is about to come. This will prevent injury and allow you to exercise more effectively.

Since I'm highlighting the importance of blood, I would also like to highlight the importance a healthy diet in keeping the organs that transport our blood functioning correctly: our veins, arteries and heart. If they get blocked up or put under too much pressure from a build up of unhealthy fat cells, you die. That's it. No ifs or buts, it's game over.

Breathing

Breathe in as deep as you can, slowly, fill your lungs up, and hold it for three full seconds then slowly exhale, completely emptying your lungs. How does that feel? How you breathe is a good indication of your health, considering it's something we need our bodies to do constantly to stay alive I would be deeply concerned if I began to encounter problems with it.

Due to the higher demand for oxygen and nutrients throughout the body when we exercise, our hearts beat faster to pump more blood around the body and the rate at which we breathe increases to meet the higher demand for oxygen. This is why it is so important to breathe deeply, regularly and in a controlled manner when exerting yourself with weightlifting. Holding your breath and tensing up is a recipe for disaster. The most effective and common way of breathing while weightlifting is to breathe out for the lift or exerting part of an exercise and then breathe in as you lower or return the weight.

It would be appropriate to mention now that you shouldn't drink carbonated drinks while exercising, whether it's water, soda or an energy drink. This is because your body is already trying to pay an oxygen debt and gassy drinks full of carbon dioxide will only hinder this process. No it wouldn't kill you if you did have one, but you could exercise much more efficiently if you didn't.

TOP TIPS:

- Your muscles require FUEL to move, from your food or fat stores on your body
- The bigger your muscles the more FUEL they will burn
- Your muscles burn FUEL all day and night, during any activity (even sleeping), but burn A LOT more when exercising
- Your muscles tear when lifting weights, the repairing process takes many hours and burns EVEN MORE FUEL
- High quality food is important so your body has the best FUEL and NUTRIENTS available to repair itself
- You lose fat from all over your body at the same time

- Blood carries everything around our bodies that we need to function and stay alive
- Stretching and warming-up fills our muscles with blood and allows us to workout safely and efficiently
- Our bodies have a higher demand for OXYGEN when we exercise, so breathing deeply and regularly is important
- Avoid carbonated drinks while exercising

5. NUTRITION

Eating well, to best fuel your mind and body or completely physically transform it, can be as simple or complicated as you make it. Books and magazines, Television and the Internet all seem to be saturated with *so much* information, conflicting rules and expensive, time-consuming diets. One day you hear *this* and another you hear *that*. This avalanche of information can make the simple life-choice of eating a healthy, balanced diet very daunting, when it absolutely is NOT.

If I could only give you one piece of advice to eating the healthiest diet possible it would be: **DON'T EAT ANYTHING MAN MADE**. Preparing all of your own meals using fresh, natural food would fill your body with the highest quality fuel and a plethora of essential nutrients whilst simultaneously avoiding anything unnatural and potentially harmful from synthetic, innutritious food. Suddenly everything you eat would be something beneficial; even a burger with chips or chicken curry with rice would become natural and nutrient rich! The burger, for example, could be shaped using the leanest mince meat you can find, then grill it to remove even more fat, use a small wholemeal bun, raw tomato, lettuce and onion inside the burger, chop some potatoes (sweet potatoes if you fancy) and either bake them or cook them in a frying pan with just enough olive oil so they don't stick, add some raw spinach and peppers to the plate for a lively salad and *voila*! If you've been treating your body poorly, eating lots of low quality food and you decided to follow that advice for just one month, and didn't even exercise, you would still notice a huge physical and mental change. Though I will be going into more detail, this will always be the best advice you could ever follow to improve the quality of your diet, health and overall wellbeing.

With so many 'diets' out there, which one is 'right'? And what are my credentials to speak on the matter? As I said in the introduction I'm not a personal trainer or a nutritionist, but I *do* understand my body, the fuel I put it in and how to make myself feel great and look the way I want. The problem with the popular idea of a 'diet' is that it is something inherently temporary; it is something you begin and so something that you end as well. Even *THE 'BE RAD' BEDROOM BODY BOOK* lays out a nutritional plan to follow for 1, 2 or 3 months, which could of course be called a diet. I *am* endorsing a temporary diet as a means to lose excess fat and improve your lifestyle and wellbeing. Once you've followed this nutritional guide religiously for 1, 2 or 3 months, and have gone completely cold turkey on all the 'treats' I will be mentioning later, I hope that you would be able to implement what you have learned indefinitely, referencing this guide to inform a permanent healthy, balanced lifestyle choice.

Personally, I think this initial, very strict 1, 2 or 3 month diet – that denies you many, *many* things you may be used to – is a powerful tool in changing your mentality towards eating healthily forever. If you do stick with it, YOU **WILL** SEE AND FEEL THE RESULTS OF YOUR COMMITMENT; the physical results will speak for themselves, and your confidence, strength of character and self-respect will all reach dizzying heights. Unless you don't like feeling physically fit, breathing easily and waking up energised, you will want to continue putting the best fuel into your body for the rest of your life.

At first, it will seem as though you are being very tough on yourself, and you are, but if you have been stuck in harmful patterns it takes this **HARD WORK** to pull yourself out of them; that is what the *very* strict few months are intended to do before you start allowing yourself treats in moderation again, while still fuelling yourself with the highest quality, natural fuel and filling your body with an abundance of nutrients. The goal of this nutritional plan is to shock the body into feeling great, and it will.

Once you've finished the strict few months the key to consistently eating well so you look and feel great is to continue to **eat a balanced assortment of fresh, high quality, natural foods**. So long as you are getting all the nutrients your body needs you can eat ice cream, pizza, crisps and have alcohol, coffee and sodas **IN MODERATION**. That is *very* important, moderation; that's where people, including myself, tend to go wrong. When your entire diet consists of premade, preserved, sugar and salt filled convenience foods you are starving your body of essential fuel and instead filling it with *empty* fuel. You get all the excess calories that will be stored as fat but none of the nutrients your body needs. You will always be hungry, no matter how many chocolate bars, multi-packs of crisps and cans of fizzy drink you consume, because your body doesn't have what it needs, so it will still tell you it needs more food, and so you eat even more to stop feeling hungry. When you eat a healthy, balanced diet you don't get hunger-cravings because your body has the fuel it needs already.

Food Groups

Carbohydrates

Carbohydrates give our bodies the energy we need to think, move our muscles and keep our systems and organs functioning, without carbohydrates you are not eating a healthy diet; they are broken down by our bodies and from them we get all the simple sugars that fuel us. They can be spilt into two groups, simple and complex carbohydrates. Simple carbohydrates don't require much breaking down by our stomachs, they are 'simple', and the sugar is released into our systems quickly. Complex carbohydrates require a lot more time to break down, think of them as being more 'complicated', so the sugar takes a lot longer to be released into our systems.

A simple method of telling how complex carbohydrates like bread, past and rice are, would be the colour; light coloured pastas, rice and breads are higher in simpler sugars that are broken down quicker in the body while the darker coloured pastas, rice and breads are usually wholegrain, wholemeal or wholewheat and take longer for our bodies to break them down into simple sugars. So long as they are natural and high quality both light and dark carbohydrates can feature in a healthy diet when consumed **IN MODERATION** because they do provide fuel our bodies can use.

The simplest of simple carbohydrates would be something like fruit, the sugar is already in a simple, natural sugar form, and can be absorbed almost straight away into our bodies. A complex carbohydrate would be wholewheat pasta; it takes more time and effort for our stomach to convert this food into a simple sugar that can be carried around our bodies. Remember the importance of blood from earlier? It is the blood that will carry the simple sugar to our muscles to be used; you can imagine, putting the sugar into our bodies in the form of a sweet piece of fruit means it is ready for transportation straight away, whereas a big piece of solid, wholemeal pasta will require a lot more breaking down and converting before the simple sugar is ready for our blood to transport.

Some people, including myself when I started lifting weights, think that if you just eat lots of protein your muscles will grow. Wrong. If you are trying to increase the size of your muscles you need to consume more carbohydrates than you do protein; you need the sugars from carbohydrates for your body to be able to process the protein correctly and grow your muscles.

Protein

Protein is the building blocks of cells, it repairs damaged cells and builds muscles. You need protein as part of a healthy diet, but if you are lifting weights you need to pay extra attention to the amount of protein you are consuming to ensure you are getting enough high quality protein so your muscles repair and grow. High protein foods would be meat, eggs, nuts and seeds.

Fat

Fats are not your enemy! There are different kinds of fats and the *right* kind of fat is an essential part of a healthy diet, even a weight loss diet! Foods high in fat contain more fuel than carbohydrates and provide us with essential oils and nutrients. Let's say there are *bad* fats (saturated fats) found in cakes, sweets, fast-food, etc. and *good* fats (unsaturated and polyunsaturated fats) found in fish, nuts, seeds and many other *natural* foods. The polyunsaturated fat from a serving of walnuts is a clean, natural fat our body can easily break down and utilise, whereas the saturated fat from a deep-fried sausage in batter is unnatural and complicated, as a result parts of the saturated fat end up clogging the inside of our arteries and increasing our risk of heart conditions.

Fibre

Fibre keeps our digestive tract clean, flowing and flushed out. Wholegrain foods, fruits and vegetables are all high in fibre.
Digestive complications and conditions can occur in people who eat lots of pre-made, man-made convenience food because they contain very little fibre, no *real* substance. It is natural fibre that pushes, scrapes and cleans our insides out; man-made, artificial, synthetic food doesn't flush out our system as nature intended our food to do.

Eating To Lose Weight

Stopping eating food altogether is stupid and dangerous, long term you will obviously die, but even in the short term it is incredibly unhealthy and you can cause irreparable damage to yourself. **DO NOT THINK THAT IF YOU STOP EATING FOOD YOU WILL LOSE ALL THE FAT ON YOUR BODY**. When you don't eat food your body digests itself, both your healthy functioning muscle-mass as well as your fat stores are consumed, your bones and joints become brittle and the systems in your body kick into starvation mode. Any food you do get after this happens will be stored as fat, no matter how lean or healthy the meal is. Your body is brilliant, if you starve yourself it doesn't know when the next meal will be coming, so looking out for your survival it stores everything as fat in case it needs the energy in the future if you continue to starve.

Hopefully you are beginning to see your body as the machine it is, constantly burning fuel and needing more fuel. As with any machine, it needs to be regularly fuelled and **WHEN** we put fuel into our bodies is *very* important. The best possible way to fuel your body, so it is using and storing its fuel most efficiently, is to eat little and often. Eat regular smaller meals and healthy snacks, as opposed to skipping breakfast, having a junk-food lunch and a huge, overloading dinner (or any other such irregular eating pattern). You could have three meals with two substantial snack breaks in between, suddenly an erratic day of starvation and calorie overload would be turned into five small meals a day. Your body would use the energy from one food intake, but before it kicked into starvation mode it would be time for the next food intake; with appropriate portion sizes you won't be storing any excess food as fat and you won't get hungry or lack energy because of the shorter wait before you get another source of fuel.

Eating to put weight on or lose weight is as simple as eating more or less food. If you put more fuel into your body than it needs, the excess will get stored as fat and your weight increases. If you put less fuel into body than it needs, your body will turn to your fat stores for the extra fuel and your weight decreases.

With regards to substantially increasing your muscle mass, you would have to consume an excess amount of high quality fuel, as well as regularly lifting heavy weights; if your body is turning to your fat stores for fuel then you are not getting enough fuel to greatly increase the size of your muscles. You won't put on a *massive* amount of muscle mass on a weight loss nutrition plan, like the one in this book. If you follow the meal plans and exercises in this book your muscles will get bigger, stronger, denser and *appear* much larger as the excess fat disappears from your body; but you won't be adding 6 inches to your arms or gaining 20kg of muscle.

Eating Around Training

When you consume food, blood rushes to your stomach so all the correct processes to break it down can occur. If you start exercising straight after eating a big meal all the blood needed in your stomach rushes to your muscles to make sure they can function, the food in your stomach that still needs breaking down won't be processed because there is no blood to provide the organs there with what they need to do their job, this food is then rejected by the body in the quickest way possible and you would be sick (expelling the food from your body). This is why you should **never** train on a full stomach.

Of course we need to have fuel in our bodies so we can exercise to the best of our abilities, so it is important to allow enough time for our bodies to break down anything we have eaten and have the simple sugars from that food readily available for our muscles to use. Depending on what you eat, both the contents and size of a meal, the length of time to wait before exercising will vary. If you eat a large solid meal containing, for example, potatoes, a chicken breast and vegetables, you should wait at least **two hours** before doing any strenuous exercise; this is because your stomach requires a lot of blood as well as the necessary amount of time to break this large amount of complicated food down, ready for your body to use. If you had only eaten a piece of fruit, you could wait **45 minutes** before exercising, not only because of the much smaller amount of food in your stomach, but also because the simple sugars will be almost instantly available for your body to use.

After exercising, especially exercising with weights, it is also important to consume food so your body can refuel and repair itself. Again, we must observe the process of the blood in our bodies to ensure we keep it running efficiently. During exercise your muscles get pumped full of blood to fuel the actions they are carrying out, after exercising it is important to allow this higher blood flow to continue there for a short time so our muscles get everything they need to recuperate and we don't injure ourselves. A compromise has to be reached that allows us to eat more food and refuel our body after a workout, but also keeps the blood flowing to our muscles rather than our stomach. For this reason there are two stages to eating after a workout.

The first would be to eat a source of simple sugar and easily digestible source of protein **5 – 20 minutes** after working out; for me this would usually be a piece of fruit and whey protein shake with semi-skimmed milk. The piece of fruit has the simplest of sugars readily available, there is also simple sugar present in the milk, the powdered protein and liquid protein in the milk again require only a small amount of blood for our bodies to absorb them. These easily absorbed sources of nutrients and fuel ensure that our muscles remained pumped with blood so they can warm down and repair effectively. This quick intake of fuel should be enough to restore your energy levels before the second stage of eating after a workout.

The second stage would be **40 minutes** after a workout, not earlier and try not to wait much longer, and at this stage you should consume a substantial, solid meal containing both a source of carbohydrate and source of protein; rice with chicken breast and spinach, for example. After pushing your body to its limit you would have used up all of your readily available sources of fuel and your muscles and organs are crying out for more. **YOU HAVE TO EAT SOMETHING AFTER A WORKOUT** if you want your muscles to get stronger, your body to repair itself and generally keep your organs and systems functioning healthily. Waiting 40 minutes should be enough time to shower and prepare some food; which could also be done while consuming your simple sources of fuel 5 – 20 minutes after a workout. This 40 minutes also allows plenty of time for the blood to finish refuelling and warming down the muscles, before it rushes to your stomach to break down and absorb the solid food you are now putting in.

These are what I would call the *most efficient guidelines*, don't beat yourself up if you deviate slightly; everyone's lives are different and I don't expect you to monitor yourself with a stopwatch, but adhere to them as best you can to maximise your results.

TOP TIPS:

- **BEST ADVICE: Don't eat anything manmade**
- **Prepare all your own meals from lean and natural food sources**
- **'Diet' knowing that you are teaching yourself to fuel your body as healthily as possible before beginning a new, much healthier, balanced lifestyle**
- **Everything *IN MODERATION***
- **You will still feel hungry after bingeing on junk food because your body DOESN'T HAVE WHAT IT NEEDS**

- Eating a healthy diet stops hunger-cravings because your body has what it needs
- Carbohydrates and fats provide energy, protein repairs cells and fibre keeps our digestive tract flushed out
- A healthy diet would contain food from each of the different groups
- Simple carbohydrates contain quickly absorbed sugars, whereas complex carbohydrates take longer to break down into absorbable sugars
- **DO NOT SKIP MEALS OR STOP EATING ALTOGETHER**
- Eat little and often to constantly refuel your body
- Don't exercise on a full stomach
- Wait 2 hours after eating a substantial meal before exercising
- Wait 45 minutes after eating some fruit, or other easily absorbed fuel source, before exercising
- Eat something simple and easily absorbed 5 – 20 minutes after a workout
- Eat a substantial meal 40 minutes after a workout

6. THE 'BE RAD' NUTRITION PLAN

I usually live a balanced lifestyle and eat a healthy range of food, still allowing myself the occasional treat, *but*... at the end of 2015 I spent a couple of months living to absolute excess. For whatever reasons I had become dissatisfied and lazy; I got drunk every other night, I lived off takeaways, fast food and microwave burgers, I became nocturnal and ashamed to see people during the day. My life had slipped into a *very* dangerous, unhealthy downward spiral. Before coming into the New Year I decided I was going to put all of the knowledge I had accumulated in my life into practice for the next 3 months, to hit the reset switch on my body and make up for the damage I may have done filling myself with such poor quality food, not exercising and drinking so much alcohol. So I designed myself the ultimate 3-month healthy living plan, both what to eat and how to exercise at home, and it is this 3-month plan – which called on my years of knowledge and practical experience to design – that I am sharing with you. Feel free to follow this plan for 1, 2, 3 or as many months as you wish, following only the nutrition plan or only the exercise plan, or both; but the more you do and the longer you stick to it the more incredible your results will be. It will probably be the strictest diet you've ever encountered before, but if you commit to it *completely* the results it will yield, both internally and externally, will also be the most impressive you've ever encountered. So without any further ado, I present to you...

THE 'BE RAD' NUTRITION PLAN

FOR THE WHOLE THREE MONTHS YOU ARE ABSOLUTELY NOT ALLOWED ANY OF THE FOLLOWING:

- **ALCOHOL**
- **ENERGY DRINKS, CAFFEINATED DRINKS, SUGARY FIZZY DRINKS (SODAS) or FRUIT JUICES**
- **FAST FOOD or TAKEAWAYS**

Advice on Adjusting to Life Without These

Though I'm unaware of what your relationship with these

food and beverage items is like, I don't doubt that this will be one of the hardest parts of this diet, if not *the* hardest; it was for me when I began.

Alcohol is basically a poison that stops your cells communicating correctly. That **HAS** to go, but don't worry, you can have it again, *in moderation*, once you've completing your tough, life-changing initiation into healthy living. You can buy non-alcoholic beer, but do make sure it is *completely* alcohol-free; some say alcohol-free when in fact they have 0.5% or 0.05% alcohol still in them. Alcohol-free beer with 0.0% alcohol is available and once it's been chilled in a fridge, the brand I found at least, tastes just as good as the real thing. With regards to the ingredients it only contained, water, hops, barley and wheat, nothing sinister and low in calories; **but you can only allow yourself a couple of bottles at the end of every two weeks of this diet you complete.**

Consuming alcohol is such a massive part of society and culture, so don't be surprised if people turn their noses up at you, but don't succumb to peer pressure; what they think is irrelevant, be strong in yourself, **YOU ARE INVESTING IN YOUR FUTURE, YOUR HEALTH AND YOUR LIFE!**

Energy drinks, sodas, sugary drinks and fruit juices are all loaded with huge amounts of sugar and unnatural chemicals. They've got to go as well. Diet sodas also contain a host of unnatural chemicals and sweeteners, so they have to go as well. **As a reward system you may have one can of diet soda at the end of each month of this diet you complete**, though I didn't.

Caffeinated drinks can send your mood and energy levels up and down, and when bought from commercial coffee shops usually contain **HUGE** amounts of sugar as well. So they've got to go as well.

Carbonated drinks leech your bones, making them brittle. If you consume sparkling water, do so *IN MODERATION*.

Hopefully abstaining from fast food and takeaways goes without saying. NO FAST FOOD CHAINS, DRIVE-THROUGHS, KEBABS, PIZZAS, FISH AND CHIPS OR ANY OTHER SORT OF INSTANTLY PREPARED HOT FOOD. If you go to a restaurant make sure anything you eat falls within the guidelines for meals I will set out momentarily. Don't invent yourself a loophole by 'dining in' at fast food 'restaurants' because you would only be cheating yourself, undermining your entire diet and all your hard work. If you have read this far *I know* that you know the difference between a fast food 'restaurant' and an actual *restaurant*.

You will be refusing yourself a lot of other things on this diet, so much in fact I will now only be referring to what you *will* be consuming. If you slip up and have something slightly off my diet plan it shouldn't completely waste all your hard work, so long as you don't let it happen again, **BUT THESE THINGS: ALCOHOL, CAFFEINATED DRINKS, SUGARY DRINKS, SODAS AND FAST FOOD** must **NOT** be consumed if you desire change and are taking this, and yourself, seriously.

<u>THE RULES:</u>

- DRINK AT LEAST 2 LITRES OF WATER A DAY
- PREPARE ALL YOUR OWN MEALS
- HAVE ONE MEAT-FREE DAY EVERY TWO WEEKS

<u>WHAT YOU WILL ONLY BE CONSUMING:</u>

- FRUIT
- VEGETABLES
- MEAT (INCLUDING FISH)
- EGGS
- NUTS (Walnuts or Almonds)
- SEEDS (Sunflower or Pumpkin Seeds)
- PEANUT BUTTER (100% Peanuts, NO ADDITIVES)
- HONEY (NO ADDITIVES)
- WHOLEMEAL PITTA BREAD
- SEMI-SKIMMED MILK
- WATER (Tap or bottled)
- CAFFEINE-FREE FRUIT TEAS and GREEN TEA
- WHEY PROTEIN POWDER (A brand with no added sugar and purest protein)
- OLIVE OIL FOR COOKING
- REDUCED FAT HUMMUS

<u>Food Preparation Guide</u>

Earlier I mentioned how efficient my nutrition plan is, that was not only with regards to fuelling and repairing your body, but also with regards to its real world application. I live a very busy life, so I keep my meal preparation times and the amount of washing up I create to an unbeatable minimum. Mainly because the only two things you will be cooking will be the meat and eggs, EVERYTHING ELSE IS EATEN RAW.

To cook all of the meat you will be consuming you should grill it in an electric grill that drains the fat away from the meat. These small electric grills are available everywhere and at very affordable prices; they easily fit on worktops or can be stored in a cupboard once they have cooled down. This is an essential piece of kit that you need in order to make sure the meat you are consuming is as lean as possible. Once a week you may cook a portion of meat in a frying pan, with the minimum amount of olive oil needed so that it doesn't stick, all the other meat you consume must be grilled and drained of fat. Also, before cooking any meat you should remove all the skin and cut off any noticeable lumps of fat or grizzle.

You should purchase the leanest cuts of meat possible, and avoid mincemeat. Skinless and boneless chicken breast is quick to grill, high in protein, low in fat and can be kept in the fridge for the following day, I eat at least one a day (so if you like chicken then you're in for a good time!).

All of the fruit and vegetables will be consumed raw, for this reason it is important to wash them all with water before you do so. You can follow your own personal preferences for peeling or eating the skins of certain fruits and vegetables, such as cucumber, carrots and apples. Personally I don't peel any, this saves even more time. The amount of preparation my vegetables require is negligible; I cut the end off my carrots, cut the seed-covered centre out of my peppers and generally chop things into bite-sized chunks if I feel like it. Don't buy anything frozen, everything should be FRESH. The only tinned produce you may consume is sweetcorn, though make sure it contains no additives.

Pre-made sauces can contain lots of sugar and salt, so we won't be using any of them, *ever*. If want to sprinkle herbs or pepper on to some of your meals then feel free to do so, but sauces are a no-go. You may sprinkle one pinch of salt on one meal a day if you so wish, but no more than that.

Meal Guide

In this diet we will be consuming **main meals** and **snacks**; the number of which in each day and when we eat them will depend on your lifestyle and when you fit your workouts into that lifestyle; as a general rule we will consume **3 MAIN MEALS** with **2 SNACKS** between them every day. The general structure of a **MAIN MEAL** and **SNACK** would be:

MAIN MEAL: 1 PROTEIN PORTION, 2 or 3 VEGETABLE PORTIONS and 1 FRUIT PORTION

SNACK: 1 FRUIT PORTION or 1 NUT SERVING or 1 SEED SERVING

Portion size is completely relative; the muscles in your body may require more or less fuel than mine. There is no way I could write a perfect nutritional plan with exact portion sizes that will cater to everyone's requirements (the same will apply to the amount of weight and number of exercises detailed later on). I am a 5'8" man who weighs 12.5 stone; I consider myself of average height and average build, though I possess slightly more muscle mass than average, which of course I've worked for and am unashamedly proud of (AND SOON YOU WILL BE JUST AS PROUD OF YOURS AS WELL!). I'm going to be telling you exactly what I eat and from that, you can eat slightly more or slightly less. Don't forget it has taken me a long time to understand my body, so don't be afraid to experiment with your portion sizes initially.

With regards to the particular meat or vegetable choices listed in the meal plans you are about to read, feel free to change them to whatever you want. It is important to include a variety of colours of fruit and vegetables to fill yourself with a range of nutrients, so experiment and have fun with it! I have listed chicken and tuna wherever a portion of protein is required, but any other equally substantial portion of protein would be adequate. It is important the meat remains as lean as possible. Also, you should **only have red meat a maximum of twice a month** and you should **only eat the same type of fish a maximum of twice a week**.

To cook my eggs I crack them into the pan and stir all the yokes and egg whites together into a light yellow mixture (as if you were going to make an omelette) but as the egg begins to cook I continue to stir, chop and mix the egg into scrambled egg. You are more than welcome to turn the multiple eggs that will be in the pan into an omelette if you can, but due to the larger number of eggs we will be using it may be harder than you are used to.

Eggs are full of protein, but the **egg yoke is also high in cholesterol**, for this reason you should **only have a maximum of 2 egg yokes a day**; it is perfectly healthy to have more egg whites. If you haven't separated egg yokes from egg whites before it is very simple to do, once you've cracked the egg simply keep the two halves of the shell close together and allow the egg white to slide through the gap while keeping the yoke trapped inside the two halves.

If you are following this plan for 3-months then during the first month you will follow the **STAGE 1 MEAL PLAN** and for the second and third months you will follow the **STAGE 2 MEAL PLAN**. If you are following this plan for less than 3-months you should follow the **STAGE 2 MEAL PLAN** straight away. The only difference between them is that in the **STAGE 1 MEAL PLAN** you will have **one regular wholemeal pitta bread** with some of the main meals, but in the **STAGE 2 MEAL PLAN** this pitta bread is completely removed from the plan. This means that the only carbohydrates will be coming from natural sugars in the fruit, vegetables, honey and milk.

The days listed in the meal plan are not in any particular order you have to follow; if you workout on a certain day, in the morning or evening, follow the corresponding plan, or if you don't workout follow the **NON-WORKOUT DAY** plan, or if it is your fortnightly meat-free day then follow the **MEAT-FREE DAY** plan.

STAGE ONE MEAL PLAN (Month 1)

NON-WORKOUT DAY

Main Meal 1: 2 Whole Eggs + 1 Egg Whites, 1 Wholemeal Pitta Bread, 1 Portion of Cherry Tomatoes, 1 Portion of Baby Spinach Leaves

Snack 1: 1 Banana

Main Meal 2: 1 Tin Tuna, Half a Cucumber, 1 Apple

Snack 2: 1 Serving of Walnuts

Main Meal 3: 1 Chicken Breast, 1 Wholemeal Pitta Bread, 2 Carrots, Half a Red Pepper, 1 Portion of Red Grapes

MEAT-FREE DAY

Main Meal 1: 1 Whole Egg + 2 Egg Whites, 1 Wholemeal Pitta Bread, 1 Portion of Cherry Tomatoes, 1 Portion of Baby Spinach Leaves

Snack 1: 1 Banana

Main Meal 2: Half a small pot of Hummus, 2 Carrots, Half a Cucumber, 1 Apple

Snack 2: 1 Serving of Walnuts

Main Meal 3: 1 Whole Egg + 2 Egg Whites, 1 Wholemeal Pitta Bread, Half a Green Pepper, 1 Portion of Broccoli, 1 Portion of Red Grapes

WORKING OUT IN THE MORNING

Snack 1: Half a teaspoon of Peanut Butter or Honey, 1 Clementine

EXERCISE (AT LEAST 45 MINUTES AFTER 'Snack 1')

Snack 2 (5-20 Minutes Post-Workout): 1 Scoop of Whey Protein Powder with 400ml Semi-skimmed Milk, 1 Banana

Main Meal 1 (40 Minutes Post-Workout): 1 Chicken Breast, 1 Wholemeal Pitta Bread, 2 Carrots, 1 Portion of Cherry Tomatoes, 1 Portion of Baby Spinach Leaves

Main Meal 2: 1 Tin of Tuna, Half a Cucumber, 1 Apple

Main Meal 3: 2 Whole Eggs + 4 Egg Whites, 1 Wholemeal Pitta Bread, 1 Portion of Sweetcorn, Half a Green Pepper, 1 Portion of Red Grapes

WORKING OUT IN THE EVENING

Main Meal 1: 2 Whole Eggs + 4 Egg Whites, 1 Wholemeal Pitta Bread, Half a Green Pepper, 1 Portion of Red Grapes

Main Meal 2: 1 Tin of Tuna, Half a Cucumber, 1 Apple

Snack 1: 1 Serving of Walnuts, 1 Clementine

EXERCISE (AT LEAST 45 MINUTES AFTER 'Snack 1')

Snack 2 (5-20 Minutes Post-Workout): 1 Scoop of Whey Protein Powder with 400ml Semi-skimmed Milk, 1 Banana

Main Meal 3 (40 Minutes Post-Workout): 1 Chicken Breast, 1 Wholemeal Pitta Bread, 2 Carrots, 1 Portion of Cherry Tomatoes, 1 Portion of Baby Spinach Leaves

STAGE TWO MEAL PLAN (Months 2 + 3)

NON-WORKOUT DAY

Main Meal 1: 2 Whole Eggs + 2 Egg Whites, 1 Portion of Cherry Tomatoes, 1 Portion of Baby Spinach Leaves, 1 Clementine

Snack 1: 1 Banana

Main Meal 2: 1 Tin Tuna, 1 Apple

Snack 2: 1 Serving of Walnuts

Main Meal 3: 1 Chicken Breast, Half a Cucumber, 1 Carrot, Half a Red Pepper, 1 Portion of Red Grapes

MEAT-FREE DAY

Main Meal 1: 1 Whole Egg + 2 Egg Whites, 1 Portion of Cherry Tomatoes, 1 Portion of Baby Spinach Leaves

Snack 1: 1 Banana

Main Meal 2: Half a small pot of Hummus, 1 Carrot, Half a Cucumber, 1 Apple

Snack 2: 1 Serving of Walnuts

Main Meal 3: 1 Whole Egg + 2 Egg Whites, Half a Green Pepper, 1 Portion of Broccoli, 1 Portion of Red Grapes

WORKING OUT IN THE MORNING

Snack 1: Half a teaspoon of Peanut Butter or Honey, 1 Clementine

EXERCISE (AT LEAST 45 MINUTES AFTER 'Snack 1')

Snack 2 (5-20 Minutes Post-Workout): 1 Scoop of Whey Protein Powder with 300ml Semi-skimmed Milk, 1 Banana

Main Meal 1 (40 Minutes Post-Workout): 1 Chicken Breast, 1 Carrot, 1 Portion of Cherry Tomatoes, 1 Portion of Baby Spinach Leaves

Main Meal 2: 1 Tin of Tuna, Half a Cucumber, 1 Apple

Main Meal 3: 2 Whole Eggs + 4 Egg Whites, 1 Portion of Sweetcorn, Half a Green Pepper, 1 Portion of Red Grapes

WORKING OUT IN THE EVENING

Main Meal 1: 2 Whole Eggs + 4 Egg Whites, 1 Portion of Cherry Tomatoes, 1 Portion of Baby Spinach Leaves, 1 Portion of Red Grapes

Main Meal 2: 1 Tin of Tuna, Half a Cucumber, 1 Apple

Snack 1: 1 Serving of Walnuts, 1 Clementine

EXERCISE (AT LEAST 45 MINUTES AFTER 'Snack 1')

Snack 2 (5-20 Minutes Post-Workout): 1 Scoop of Whey Protein Powder with 300ml Semi-skimmed Milk, 1 Banana

Main Meal 3 (40 Minutes Post-Workout): 1 Chicken Breast, 1 Carrot, Half a Green Pepper, 1 Portion of Sweetcorn

What Time Should I Eat?

When we eat is also important, especially in this plan that relies on natural sugar hits from fruit and vegetables. As a general rule on **non-workout days** leave around 5-6 hours between main meals and have the snacks at the midpoint between them. On **workout days** leave around 4 hours between the consecutive main meals and follow the aforementioned rules regarding eating the snacks before and after training. Let me show you how this plays out in reality and what time I was consuming my different meals and snacks:

NON-WORKOUT DAY
Main Meal 1: 8:00 am
Snack 1: 10:30 am
Main Meal 2: 1:30 pm
Snack 2: 4:45 pm
Main Meal 3: 7:00 pm

WORKING OUT IN THE MORNING
Snack 1: 8:00 am
EXERCISE 45 MINUTES LATER (Exercising for 1 – 1.5 hours)
Snack 2 (5-20 Minutes Post-Workout): 10:30 am
Main Meal 1 (40 Minutes Post-Workout): 11:10 am
Main Meal 2: 3:30 pm
Main Meal 3: 8:00 pm

WORKING OUT IN THE EVENING
Main Meal 1: 8:00 am
Main Meal 2: 12:30 Midday
Snack 1: 4:30 pm
EXERCISE 45 MINUTES LATER (Exercising for 1 – 1.5 hours)
Snack 2 (5-20 Minutes Post-Workout): 7:10 pm
Main Meal 3 (40 Minutes Post-Workout): 7:50 pm

This is a very generalised explanation of how I ate and exercised around my busy working life; my meal times varied constantly, as did my workload and the amount of travelling I had to do. Some days I'd have 4 snacks and 2 main meals, or 4 main meals and 1 snack, some days I ate 2 hours after one meal and other days I went 5 hours without eating anything. I couldn't stick rigidly to this plan and I wouldn't expect you to be able to either. What is important is the regularity and leaving those gaps between meals for your body to use the fuel it has. It's a very adaptable plan, but if you are new to all this then try to stick as close to it as possible.

Healthy Treats

Sparkling water with a couple of slices of lemon or cucumber in it is incredibly refreshing; you could have a glass of this every other day if you wanted to. Remember, excess consumption of carbonated drinks can leech minerals from our bones so drink sparkling water *IN MODERATION*.

Caffeine-free fruit teas and green tea I usually have later in the day to ease myself into a relaxed evening, but you're free to have them at any time. Of course have no milk or sugar with them, but still only drink them occasional, allowing yourself a maximum of two cups a day. This way you can view them as a real treat, and the flavours I have found are brilliant: pina colada, apple and pear, lemon and ginger, honey and vanilla.

Olives, avocado, sunflower seeds and pumpkin seeds are all high in *good* fats and personally I find them all very tasty. They go with any of the main meals perfectly. Only use one of them on any one-day though; again keeping them as a treat item. Sprinkle them amongst the vegetables or stir them into the scrambled egg.

If you have a juicer feel free make yourself a freshly pressed juice for breakfast on the days you are training in the morning. Keep it at a ratio of around 60% vegetables and 40% fruit, and consume a maximum of 500ml.

Chopped hazelnuts are delicious; something about chopped nuts, their surface area and your taste buds means there's a real taste explosion when you eat them. Every now and again you can swap the walnut servings with a serving of chopped hazelnuts, provided you like hazelnuts that is!

Getting Into A Routine

Eventually I developed a variety of routines with my workouts, preparing my meals, any cleaning up and even the food shopping. It all helped me plan my days so I could live, work, exercise and eat comfortably. It only takes a little bit of thinking and adapting, but once you get into your own routine you will find that you have more spare time, you're *much* less anxious about your new lifestyle shift and **YOU WILL FEEL IN CONTROL OF YOURSELF AND YOUR LIFE**. It might sound like a false hope being dangled in front of you, "Oh, if you eat these vegetables you're going to become super confident!" No, no, no… this *very* strict nutritional plan is going to test you, *every part of you*, your personality, your dedication, your willpower. Every day is going to be a battle, a battle that *you will win*, and with each *daily* victory you **will** begin to feel stronger, prouder and more sure of yourself.

This otherworldly strength of character, that I have now grown accustomed to having, will come in time; and that's only from committing to this nutrition plan… if you couple this with what is coming in **THE 'BE RAD' BEDROOM WORKOUT PLAN** … well… you may very well become the *BEST **YOU** YOU'VE EVER BEEN*.

7. MUSCLES OF THE BODY

When people first start thinking about lifting weights they often only think about their arms and chest; these muscles being the most prominent on muscled individuals while wearing a well-fitted t-shirt, so logically they must require the most attention, right? Wrong. For a truly healthy body that allows you to work out properly and looks balanced, you need to work out every muscle in your body. Once you've been training a while then you can begin to focus on weaker areas if you identify any, but initially you have to wake-up and strengthen your entire body, not just the bits that stand out in a t-shirt.

It is important to understand which muscle groups are responsible for which movements, with this knowledge we can determine which exercises will work particular parts of the body. Describing the intricacies of the muscles we have is far more complex than simply stating something like 'the bicep is a lump on the arm.' If we take the bicep for example, a bodybuilder would consider it having four parts: inner, outer, upper and lower. They carefully monitor and develop the length, thickness and height; and different exercises can be used to target specific parts of the bicep. There is a complex science to every part of training and nutrition, and it can be very off putting for those new to it, so for the sake of *THE 'BE RAD' BEDROOM BODY BOOK*, I will be keeping it as simple as possible while still delivering to you the best, no-nonsense advice. To develop the strongest, fullest looking muscles possible my workouts include exercises that target each part of the different muscle groups. Any exercises or actions mentioned here are explained, with images, in the *Exercises* section.

The easiest breakdown of the muscle groups we will be working on would be: **CHEST, SHOULDERS, BACK, TRICEPS, BICEPS** and **CORE (ABDOMINALS)**. Below you will find some very simplified diagrams which highlight these different muscle groups.

Chest

The chest is made up of slabs of muscle called pectorals, which we can consider having an upper, lower, inner and outer part. The chest is involved in lifting and pushing exercises when your body is positioned horizontally; so any form of press-up or pushing weights upwards as you lay parallel with the floor.

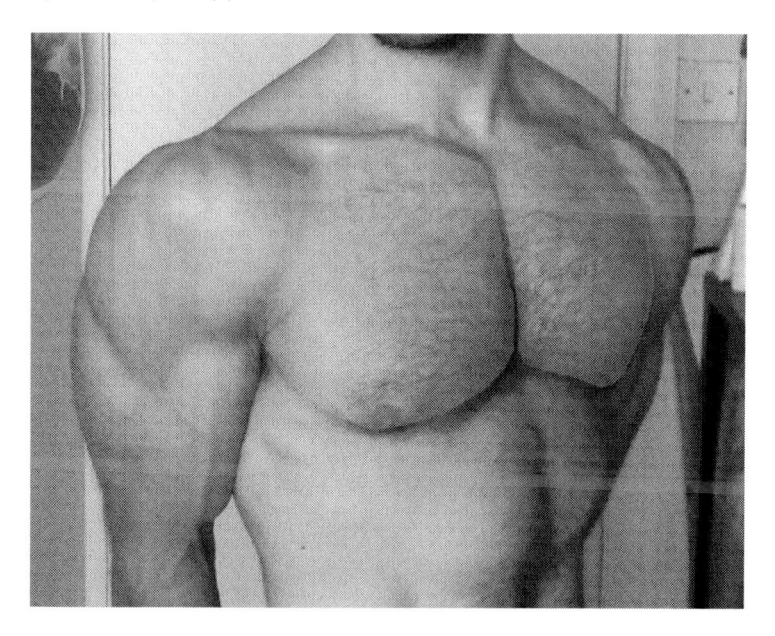

Shoulders

The shoulders are made up of a number of different muscles. Picture the curvature of the muscle on your shoulder, it is almost spherical, we can divide that sphere into three parts: the front, side and rear deltoids (named for their position on the shoulder). There is also the trapezius muscle – or 'traps' as many people shorten it to – which are the large triangular muscles on your upper back, between the corners of your shoulders that connect to your neck. The shoulders are involved in any vertical pushing or lifting exercises (pushing the weight above your head as your body is upright). They are also involved when raising weights to shoulder height or beyond without bending your arms at the elbow (which would involve the biceps or triceps).

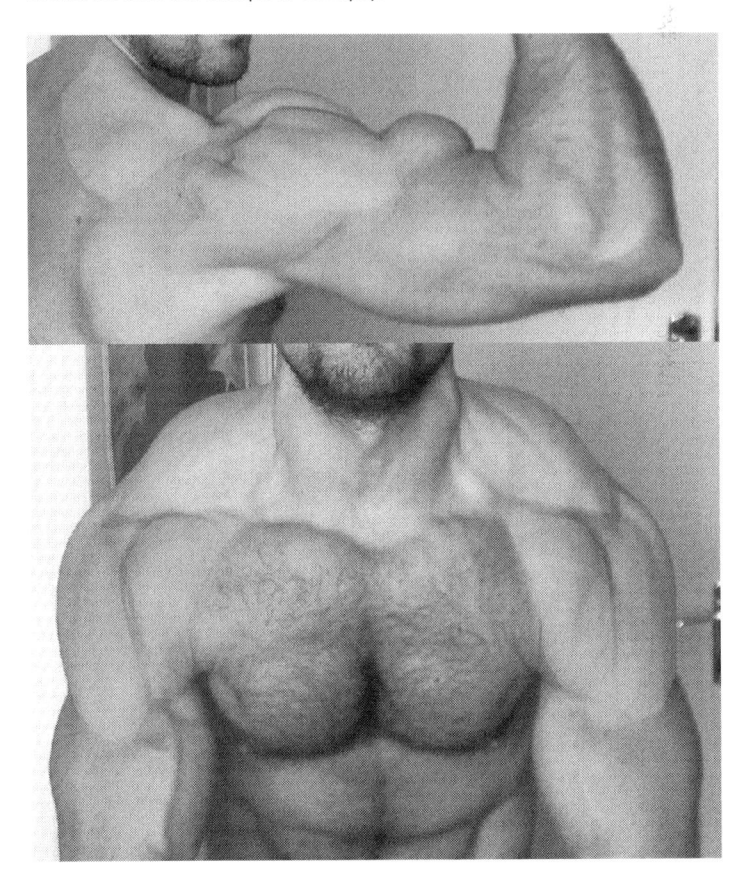

Back

There are a lot of different muscles in your back, for simplicity we will be considering the back as one large muscle, the V-shaped latissimus dorsi ('lats' for short), with a collection of smaller muscles in the upper back. The back is involved whenever pulling weight towards it, imagine the action of rowing, pulling the oar towards your body greatly involves the muscles in your back. Without a rowing machine, we can simulate this action by positioning the body horizontally and pulling the weight from the floor towards the body.

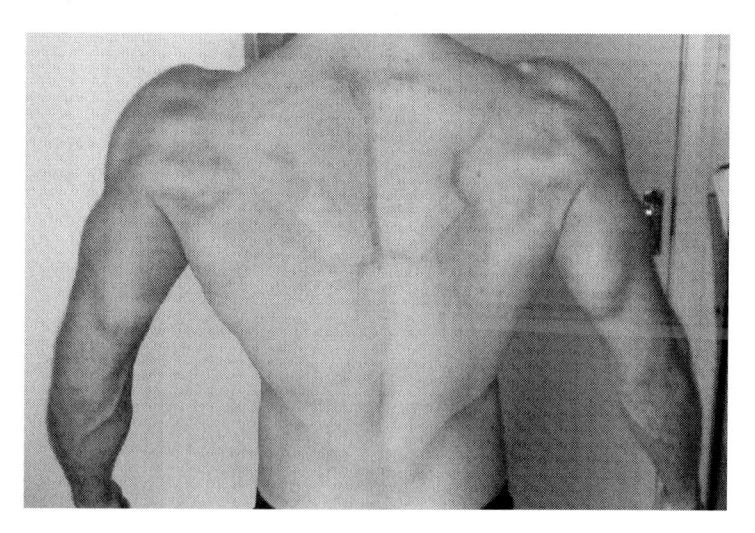

Triceps

The triceps are the horseshoe shaped muscle on the outside/rear part of the arm. People who want big arms usually focus on working out their biceps, when in fact two thirds of your upper arm is made up of the triceps! If you want bigger arms think, "Triceps, triceps, triceps!" The triceps are involved in any exercise where the exertion is due to extending the arm away from the body; whether over your head while your body is vertical or from your chest to your waist with your body horizontal. The triceps are also involved in any pressing exercises, both horizontal chest pressing and vertical shoulder pressing.

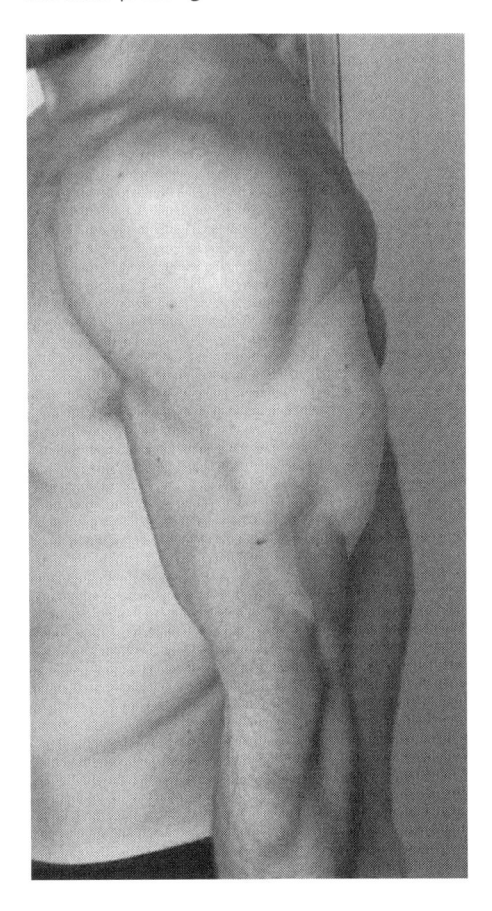

Biceps

Biceps. The first image that comes to most people's minds when they hear the words gym, muscle or flex would be that of someone bending their arm and flexing one of their biceps. Working on your biceps and filling your sleeves can be an incredible confidence booster, but don't neglect the rest of your body.

The biceps have an outer, inner, upper and lower section (referred to as 'heads'). The outer head is the outside of the bicep (on display while our arms are at our sides), the inner head is the inside of the bicep (on show with our arms above our heads), the upper head refers to the uppermost length of the bicep which connects to the shoulder and the lower head refers to the lowermost length of the bicep that connects to the inside of the elbow.

The length and height of your biceps are also good to be aware of. Some people have biceps that stretch the whole length of the upper arm and some people have a noticeable gap between the elbow and the bicep; I fall into the latter of these two groups, as you can see in the images. This is down to genetics and I'm yet to encounter any advantages or disadvantages to the different lengths of biceps other than physical appearance. I do however ensure that I include lots of exercises that activate that lower head of my bicep to keep it as strong as the rest of the muscles in my arm.

The biceps are involved in any form of curling exercise; lifting the weight from your side to your chest by bending your arm but keeping your elbow positioned at your side. Different variations of curling will work the different heads of the biceps and give them a full look (I have implemented these variations into the workouts detailed later).

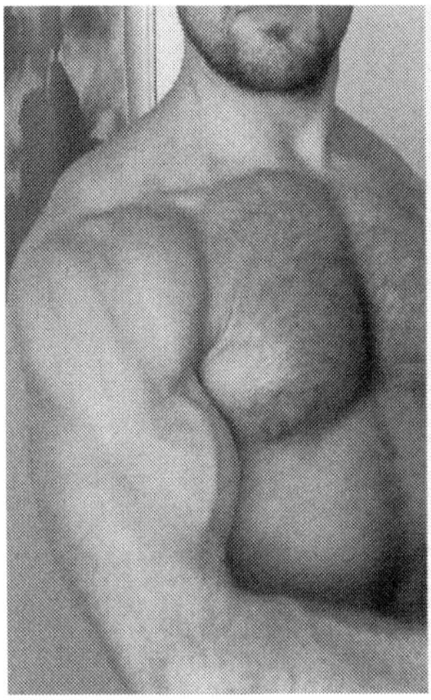

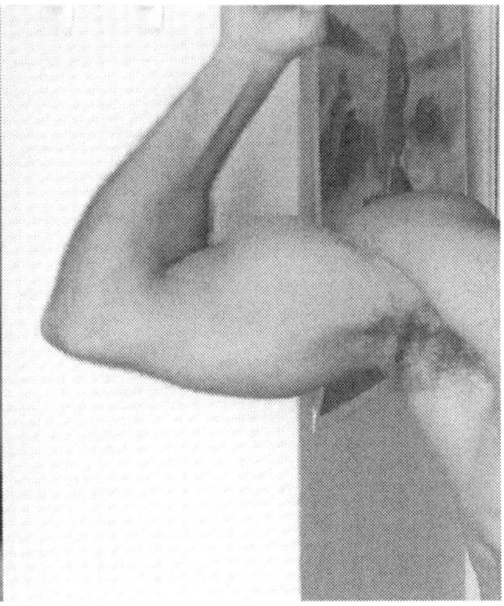

Core

By **CORE** I mean your abdominal, oblique and intercostal muscles, as well as all the muscles in your lower back, on your hips and around your waistline. This massive collection of muscles supports your spine and the centre of your body during every activity you do, which includes exercise and during day-to-day living. They are constantly being used and are therefore constantly being worked out. When you start lifting weights for the first time it is of **VITAL IMPORTANCE** you exercise and listen to the muscles in your core, and that doesn't just mean the 'six pack' abs at the front, THAT MEANS YOUR ENTIRE **CORE**. Lifting, twisting and bending, especially when there's heavy weights involved, puts a *lot* of pressure on your body, if you lift weights in a reckless manner or have very weak core strength, you **WILL** injure yourself, possibly for life. I'm not trying to scare or worry any of you, I just want to make you aware of how important not only correct, controlled workout techniques are, but also how important your **CORE** muscles are.

I workout my entire core before every weights workout, I consider this my warm-up before lifting weights; it gets the blood pumping around my entire body and I can be sure that the muscles around my lower spine and mid-section are awake and ready for action.

The muscles in your core will activate with every exercise you do, but there are exercises illustrated later that target and strengthen the individual muscles of the core.

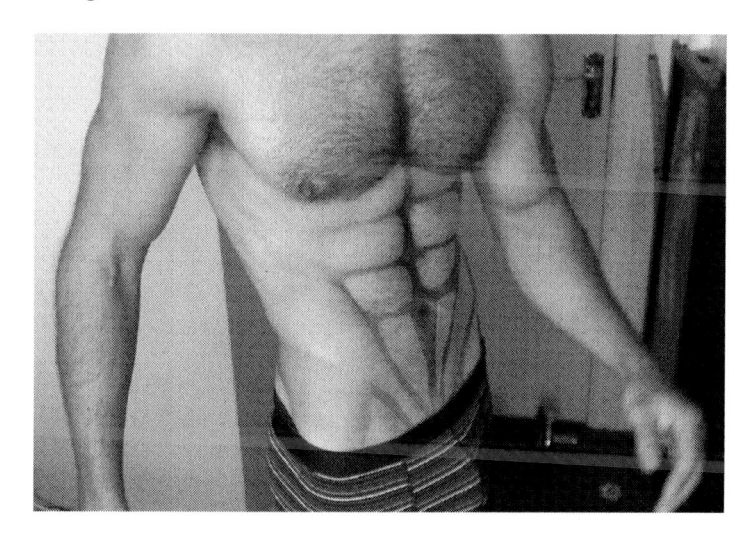

What have we missed?

This has been a *very* simplified breakdown of the muscles in your body. I'm not claiming to be a doctor or physiotherapist I simply wanted to give you enough information to make sure you understand how your body works and why my routines will as well. You could say I've missed out the forearms, or gluteus maximus (the gluts, your bum muscles), or any number of others, but my workouts do involve every muscle of the body at some point. To comment on these two examples in particular; your forearms get used all the time in most of the weight exercises, especially when we change the position of the wrist, and the gluts are involved in most of the leg and core work as well.

For everyone wondering about the muscles in your legs: Your legs contain massive and powerful muscles; the quadriceps, hamstrings and calves (amongst others). When you walk, run, use stairs, jump, swim, bend, kick, turn and even stand, the muscles in your legs are being used. As with your core, they are involved in almost every physical activity you could possibly do. Coming from someone who couldn't walk for a year and has the knees of 200 year old professional rugby player, your legs are so incredibly important and should never be taken for granted, keeping the muscles and joints in them strong, flexible and healthy will keep you more agile, mobile and fitter for longer. Due to the condition of my knees I have a particular way of ensuring the muscles in my legs remain strong, which are completely universal and not only for people with damaged joints. I promise you, if you follow my lead in how to strengthen your legs (without running, squatting or lifting heavy weights) you will feel them ache, grow and get much stronger. This will all be explained in detail in the *Exercises* section later.

Lots of the muscle groups overlap during the exercises; for example, the upper back and rear shoulders, the lower back during upper back work, triceps during any pressing exercises. Very few exercises *truly* isolate one muscle and don't involve *any* others, especially when working out at home with no gym-level equipment. The exercises and workouts featured later isolate individual muscles as much as possible but don't be surprised if you feel it all over, especially if this is your first time working out!

I think it's good to know what you are working with and where you want to go, take a moment to stretch the muscles in your body and identify what is where and how flexible you feel; look in a mirror if that makes it easier for you. Know that you made of exactly the same flesh and bone as everyone else, if you eat healthily and exercise you will *lose fat* and *build muscle*. If you follow my workouts and diets you will get a *lot* stronger and noticeably tone up in a matter of weeks. Yes, some people get better results quicker, some people have more muscle to start with, some people BLAH, BLAH, BLAH! There are no other people for **YOU** to worry about; you are only concerned with **YOU**; *your* hard work, *your* targets and *your* results!

TOP TIPS:

- **Workout and strengthen your ENTIRE BODY, not just one muscle group**
- **Even the individual muscles have different sections (heads) that should all be exercised for the fullest, strongest muscles possible**
- **Your CHEST and TRICEPS are involved in horizontal pressing exercises**
- **Your SHOULDERS and TRICEPS are involved in vertical pressing exercises**
- **Two thirds of you arms are TRICEPS**
- **Your BACK and LEGS are the largest muscles in your body**
- **Your CORE ensures stability around your spine when you bend, twist and lift**
- **Your CORE is your COMPLETE mid-section (not just the abs at the front)**

8. WEIGHT TRAINING EQUIPMENT

To perform all of the exercises in **THE 'BE RAD' BEDROOM WORKOUT PLAN** you will need these four bits of cheap equipment: **AN EXERCISE MAT, A SWISS BALL, A SET OF DUMBBELLS** and **A SET OF PRESS-UP HANDLES**.

When it comes to buying any exercise equipment or workout clothes, you don't *need* anything special or fancy. No amount of designer logos, fashion flaps or pictures of lightning bolts are going to make you work out any harder, that is up to *you*. When I went to the gym the shorts I wore cost £4 and my vest cost £2, and they lasted me over two years. Now I workout in my pants in my bedroom and don't even need a gym kit, haha! But if you're not on a budget then buy what you want, and if you like the latest workout top by a particular brand that costs £50, then go for it. Even if you are on a budget but can't stand the look of those cheap, bright red shorts you've seen, then set aside some money and pay more for ones you like. This is an incredible journey of self-discovery and self-improvement you're embarking on, so enjoy it!

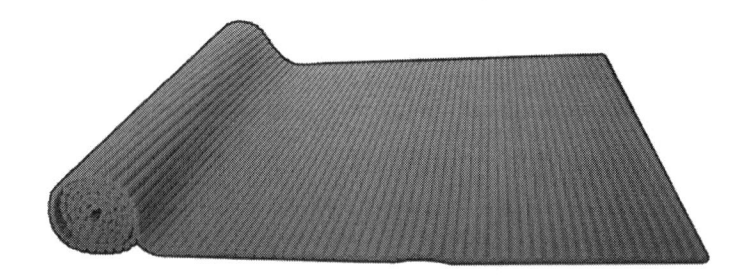

<u>EXERCISE MAT</u>

An **EXERCISE MAT** is simply a thin foam mat that measures about 6' x 3' and can easily be rolled up and stored away. This is a comfort item that rolls out on the floor to cushion your body during any floor-based exercises and stop you sweating on the carpet. It can also be folded in half and used to rest your dumbbells on between sets (to stop any banging or scratching on the floor); it will only slightly absorb any sort of impact so don't start throwing your dumbbells at it and expecting it to make your floor indestructible.

If you are happy to workout on your carpet, wooden floor or

whatever surface you have available to you, then you don't need the **EXERCISE MAT**. We won't be impacting the floor *at all* so don't think it's there to cushion your joints for any exercises; it is a comfort and hygiene item I purchased for myself, so I don't get any sweat on the floor and also so I don't get any friction burns or rashes from the coarse carpet I have in my bedroom.

These can be purchased quite cheaply these days and you really don't need anything special; it is a thin foam mat, that is all. Mine cost me £7.99 and has lasted over a year already.

SWISS BALL

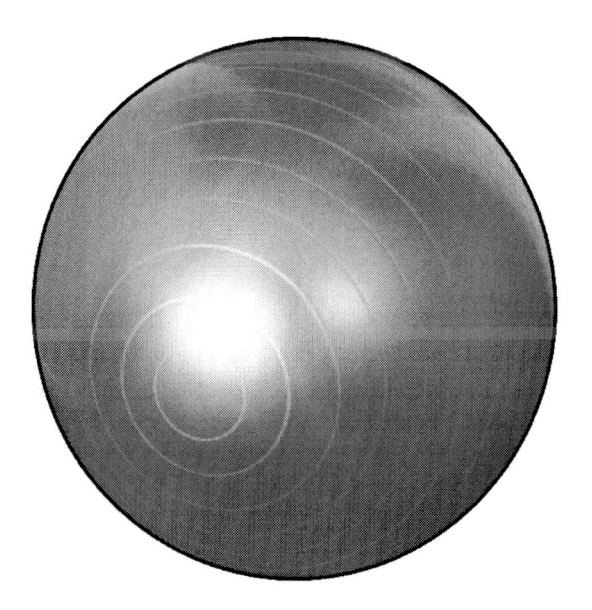

The **SWISS BALL** is large inflatable, plastic ball that we will be using for lots of our CORE exercises. It allows us to twist, bend and move our upper body in different directions to our lower body in a safe and controlled manner. Using the **SWISS BALL** to exercise we can target our abs, obliques, intercostals, hips and lower back; working out our entire core *very* effectively.

They come in a variety of different sizes, I am 5'8" and have a 55cm diameter ball. If I sit upright on the ball with my feet flat on the floor, by knees are bent at roughly a 90 degree angle, this is the right size ball for me. If you are taller than me you may need a slightly larger ball, and if you're shorter you may need a smaller ball. Again, you can find unbranded ones at very low prices, mine cost £5.49.

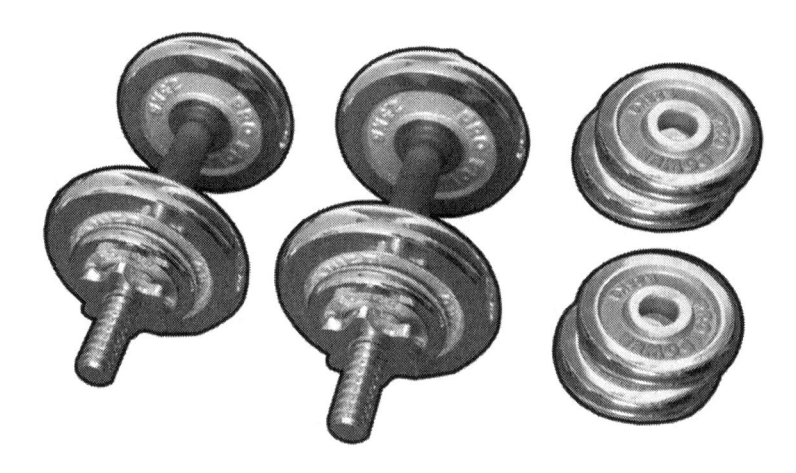

DUMBBELLS

DUMBBELLS, the most traditional and effective weight training equipment around. We will be using a set of **DUMBBELLS** for most of the main exercises in the workout plans.

The set I have is adjustable with the amount of weight on there, meaning that I only need one set but can adjust how heavy they are for the different exercises I do. You simply unscrew the large nuts from each end, attach or remove the weight plates as required, then reattach the nuts. These **DUMBBELLS** are readily available and can be found at reasonable prices. Mine cost £24.99 for a set with enough weight plates for me to complete every exercise with enough resistance. I then purchased a second set so I could have one set of dumbbells for exercises that required a heavier weight, and one set for the exercises that required less weight, just to save time on unscrewing the weights and swapping the plates over during my workouts. You can follow this example if so wish.

PRESS-UP HANDLES

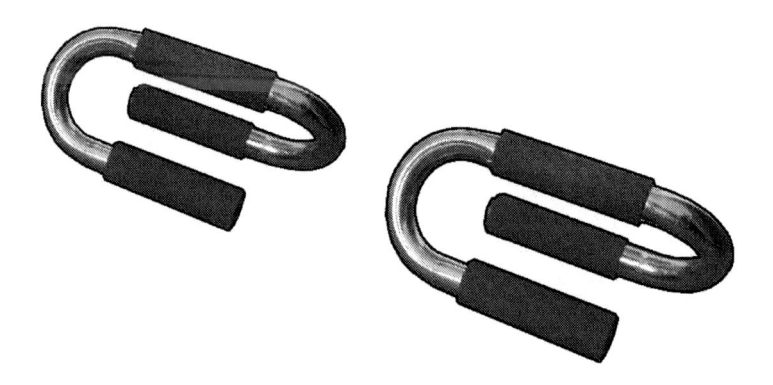

Our chest muscles are big and powerful, and without a bench press in our bedrooms we'll have to adapt in order to exercise these muscles thoroughly. We will be relying on bodyweight exercises, PRESS-UPS, of various styles. **PRESS-UP HANDLES** raise our upper bodies off the floor just enough to add a few more inches to the range of motion we can push our bodies through during our PRESS-UPS. These extra inches make a *massive* impact on the effectiveness of our PRESS-UP exercises.

Some people rest their hands on books or bricks, the effect is very much the same. I, however, prefer holding on to the curved handles to simulate the bar of the bench press; personally I feel less stress on my fingers and wrists with closed hands around the bars than I do with my hands open on a flat surface.

My **PRESS-UP HANDLES** were on sale for £4.99 and work brilliantly, after many months they still show no signs of stress or damage. Some I have seen twist and turn as you press, saying they exercise more muscles more effectively. Personally, I've never liked the thought of twisting my wrists *during* a PRESS-UP motion; I feel there is a higher risk of injury and an unnecessary amount of strain on my wrists. For these reasons **TWISTING PRESS-UP HANDLES** are not featured in any of my workouts.

9. WEIGHT TRAINING: WHAT YOU NEED TO KNOW

As I mentioned earlier, training with weights will keep your muscles repairing, growing and burning fuel for long after you've finished exercising. Once your muscles are denser and stronger, they will constantly require more fuel to function; even when you're just walking around or doing the washing up! If you do cardiovascular exercise, like swimming or running, once you've trained and built your stronger, more fuel-hungry muscles you will lose all that excess fatty-fuel on your body much, *much* quicker than you would have with cardiovascular exercise alone. Before you start, there are a few things you should know about training with weights in order to stay healthy, to exercise to the best of your ability and ensure you are getting the best results possible.

WHEN SHOULD I TRAIN?

Firstly, we will only be training **once a day**. This way your body won't be under too much pressure and you'll still have plenty of time to live your life. *When* this training session takes place is completely a matter of personal preference (though usually dictated by our work and lifestyle). Personally I prefer to work out first thing in the morning, my second choice would be late afternoon (3-4pm) and my absolute last choice would be anything around 8pm. I like waking up, feeling energised, having a piece of fruit, then waiting a short while, exercising and then eating a substantial meal to get the day started. I feel invigorated all day and know that my body will be burning fuel for a long time.

The benefit of working out in the evening would be that once you've eaten all your post-workout food you'll probably be going to sleep not long after. This means your body has all night while you sleep to use that fuel to primarily repair your muscles; you're also at no risk of straining any exhausted muscles.

Whatever time of day you do decide to train, make sure you follow the advice in the **NUTRITION** section about **EATING AROUND TRAINING**.

REPETITIONS AND SETS

REPETITIONS (shortened to **REPS**) and **SETS** are the most common way of breaking down and organising weight training; it is how all my workouts are structured so it is of vital importance you understand what they both are.

A **REPETITION** is one complete, singular exercise motion. For PRESS-UPS, starting low down, pushing your body up and then lowering yourself back to where you started, would be **ONE REPETITION** (or **REP**). For BICEP CURLS, holding a dumbbell in each hand at your side, curling them to chest height and then lowering them back to your side would be **ONE REPETITION**, and so on and so forth for all the other exercises. Each **REPETITION** should be carried out in a controlled manner and you should be consciously aware that you are using the correct form, for both your safety and to maximise the effectiveness of each **REPETITION** you perform; breathe out as you exert yourself or lift any weights and breathe in as you lower any weights or return to your original position. Remember then, a **REPETITION** is ONE COMPLETE, SINGULAR EXERCISE MOTION (and you will be doing *lots* of **REPS**!).

A **SET** is a group of **REPS** performed one after the other; so a particular number of complete, singular exercise motions performed in succession. For example, a **SET** of 10 PRESS-UPS means you perform 10 **REPS** of the complete PRESS-UP exercise.

In our workouts we will be performing numerous **SETS** of the same exercise to really get the muscles we are targeting working *hard* and growing *strong*. It is ***VERY*** important that you put the weights down, stop exerting yourself and have a short break between each **SET**, a break of around 45 seconds. This not only gives you a chance to take some deep breaths or have a sip of water, but most importantly it gives your body the time it *vitally* needs to fill your muscles with more blood and fuel so it can perform the next **SET** of exercises safely and effectively.

So how do we decide how many **REPS** there should be in a **SET**? And how many **SETS** should we be performing? The answer to both of these questions is *'enough to exhaust the muscles we are training'*. A **SET** should consist of enough **REPS** to work the muscles you are targeting to exhaustion (which will of course be affected by the amount of weight you are lifting), at the end of this exhaustive **SET** you have your 45 second break, and your body should then be ready for the next **SET**, which should contain the same number of **REPS** and again push all those muscles to exhaustion before stopping for your next 45 second break.

I can make it very simple now by letting you know that we will be performing 5 **SETS** of all the weightlifting exercises in **THE 'BE RAD' BEDROOM BODY WORKOUT PLAN**. This will be enough **SETS** so that by the final **REP** of the final **SET** you physically can't perform that exercise any more. In case you're thinking that you might be weaker or stronger than me, and performing the same number of exercises will be too hard or too easy for you, then this is where the amount of weight you are using comes into play...

The amount of weight we use to train with is completely relative, meaning that it totally depends on the individual performing the exercise. But should we use the heaviest weight we can possibly lift and do **1 REP** or barely any weight at all and do **100 REPS**? There are benefits to training at either end of the spectrum, but for **THE 'BE RAD' BEDROOM BODY WORKOUT PLAN** we will be aiming to perform between **10 - 20 REPS** in each **SET**, depending on the exercise (an exact number will be listed later); this will be enough to exhaust, strengthen and grow our muscles effectively and create a high demand for fuel in our bodies. To make sure these **10 - 20 REPS** do exhaust your muscles, you will need to find out how much weight *you* should be lifting for the most effective workout. This will take a little bit of initial experimentation: start with a very light weight you can easily lift and see how many **REPS** you can perform, allow yourself a short break, then increase the weight, note how many controlled **REPS** you can perform, have another break, then increase the weight or decrease the weight as necessary until you are only able to perform the listed number of **REPS** for **5 SETS** of that particular exercise. And there is no sense in cheating *yourself*; if you want to feel and see an incredible change then *you need to actually be working your muscles* **hard**.

For bodyweight exercises, such as the variety of PRESS-UPS and SWISS BALL SIT-UPS we will be doing, if you can't manage the number of **REPS** I originally set out for you to do, then perform as many as you can to exhaustion (even if that's only 2 or 3), have a 45 second break, and then perform as many as you can *again* until exhaustion, have another 45 second break, and then carry on until you have completed a full, exhaustive **5 SETS** of that exercise. Over time you will notice that you are growing stronger, the exercise is getting much easier, and so the number of **REPS** you have to perform until your muscles are exhausted will begin to increase; eventually you'll get to the point where you are performing hundreds of PRESS-UPS in each workout. Trust me, if you stick with it, YOU *WILL* GET THERE! On the flipside of this, if the number of **REPS** for any of the weight-free exercises is too easy, then do more; do as many as it takes to exhaust those muscles!

SUPER SETS

A **SUPER SET** is a training technique that can surprise our muscles, keep our heart rate going and exhaust our muscles even more fully; not to be overused and risk overtraining to injury or illness. A **SUPER SET** involves performing a full exhaustive **SET** of one exercise and then performing another **SET** of a different exercise straight away, WITHOUT THE USUAL 45 SECOND BREAK.

In **THE 'BE RAD' BEDROOM WORKOUT PLAN** we will count the two parts of the **SUPER SET** as only one **SET**; effectively turning the usual **5 SETS** into **10 SETS**! You can see how overusing such a technique would simply run you into the ground. It will be clearly stated later which exercises involve **SUPER SETS**.

PYRAMID SETS

A **PYRAMID SET** is a training technique which allows us to push ourselves and our muscles harder in a safe and controlled manner. It involves lowering the number of **REPS** in each progressive **SET**; which means we start with a large number of **REPS** in the 1st **SET**, then fewer in the 2nd **SET**, fewer still in the 3rd **SET**, even fewer in the 4th **SET** and then the lowest number of **REPS** in the 5th **SET**.

For example, a **PYRAMID SET** of PRESS-UPS could look like this: for the 1st **SET** you perform **20 REPS**, in the 2nd **SET** you perform **18 REPS**, in the 3rd **SET** you perform **16 REPS**, in the 4th **SET** you perform **14 REPS** and in the 5th **SET** you perform only **12 REPS**.

This is a great way to gradually increase our strength and the number of **REPS** we are able to perform over time. It is a safe and incredibly effective training tool. In **THE 'BE RAD' BEDROOM WORKOUT PLAN** we utilise **PYRAMID SETS** on the hardest exercises which target our largest muscles, again it will clearly be stated which exercises these are.

TARGETING MUSCLE GROUPS

One of the main principles of **THE 'BE RAD' BEDROOM WORKOUT PLAN** is how it targets particular muscles on one day, works them to exhaustion, then allows them days off to grow and repair while targeting other muscles the following day. After numerous meals increasing the amount of fuel available within your body and the recuperative power of a good night's sleep, you will find yourself ready to safely and effectively train the same muscles to exhaustion again very soon.

For the larger muscle groups, like those in our **chest, back** and **shoulders**, we should leave at least **48 hours** between training the same ones to total exhaustion. This allows those larger muscles the extra time they need to repair and grow. For the smaller muscles in our arms though, both **triceps** and **biceps**, we can allow **24** hours between sessions which train them to exhaustion. Since our **chest** and **shoulders** are both so closely linked and involved in heavy pressing exercises, we should also leave at least **48 hours** between sessions that train either of these large muscle groups to exhaustion.

REST & CORRECT FORM

Resting is incredibly important in making sure you remain fit and healthy when you are involved in a regular, exhaustive training routine that pushes your body to its limit; not only resting between **SETS** but also having days off from lifting weights and getting good quality, undisturbed sleep. I always aim to get at least **7 – 8 HOURS OF GOOD QUALITY SLEEP**.

You should be aiming to train **5 – 6 DAYS A WEEK**, and lifting no weights on your days off. Feel free to do any cardiovascular exercise you want on these rest days, just don't push yourself too hard.

My usual pattern for working out and resting is to **TRAIN FOR 3 DAYS IN A ROW and then HAVE A DAY OFF and then TRAIN FOR ANOTHER 3 DAYS IN A ROW**. With this schedule, which I sometimes have no choice but to deviate from, I train 5 days some weeks and 6 days other weeks. What is important is that you train regularly and get an adequate amount of rest; following this training pattern will achieve both of those goals.

Don't forget, after a weightlifting workout your muscles will be repairing themselves, so don't go diving into the swimming pool or going for a run after your weightlifting session. Any cardiovascular exercise you do on the same day as your weight training should be relatively easy going and undertaken a good few hours away from your weightlifting workout.

Working out using the **CORRECT FORM** is crucial for both your safety and to maximise your results. We will be stood upright for a large number of our weightlifting exercises, so it is EVEN MORE IMPORTANT TO KEEP OUR BODIES COMPOSED AND ALL OUR MOTIONS CONTROLLED. Move slowly through the range of motion of the exercises, **DO NOT THROW THE WEIGHTS USING YOUR BODYWEIGHT or FLING YOUR BODY FORWARD AND BACK or TWIST AT THE WAIST**. Any sudden, jerky or unnatural movements you make while holding so much extra weight on your upper body **MAY CAUSE YOU IRREPARABLE, LIFE-ALTERING DAMAGE (NAMELY, SPINAL INJURY)**.

Also, when lifting the weights off the floor and placing them back down, make sure you bend with your knees, **NOT WITH YOUR BACK**.

TOP TIPS:

- Only train once a day
- A REPETITION (or REP) is one complete, singular exercise motion
- A SET is a group of REPETITIONS performed one after the other
- Rest for 45 SECONDS between SETS
- We will be performing 5 SETS of each exercise (the number of REPS will be listed in the WORKOUT PLAN)
- The amount of weight you should be lifting should be enough to exhaust your muscles after 5 SETS (of the listed number of REPS)
- To find out how much weight exhausts your muscles start with a very light weight and increase it gradually until you can only perform the listed number of REPS
- SUPER SETS involve performing two SETS of two different exercises WITHOUT A 45 SECOND BREAK IN BETWEEN
- PYRAMID SETS involve decreasing the number of REPS in each SET you perform
- Leave at least 48 HOURS between training the

same LARGE MUSCLE GROUP to exhaustion again
- Leave at least 24 HOURS between training the same SMALLER MUSCLE GROUP to exhaustion again
- Leave at least 48 HOURS between training your CHEST and SHOULDERS to exhaustion
- Train 5 – 6 days a week
- Get 7 – 8 hours of good quality sleep
- Train for 3 days then have 1 day off from lifting weights
- Use the CORRECT FORM to prevent injury and maximise results

10. THE 'BE RAD' BEDROOM WORKOUT PLAN

Workout Structure

The overall structure of these bedroom workouts will be a short CORE training session followed by a weightlifting session which targets one large muscle group and one smaller muscle group. The CORE exercises at the start of the workout serve as the warm-up. They are performed slowly and with no weight; they primarily target the muscles in your CORE but they will wake up muscles all over your body and get your heart pumping blood to where it needs to be before you start lifting any weights.

The weightlifting sessions will focus on working out one large muscle group, either your CHEST, BACK or SHOULDERS, and then the muscles in your arms. They will consist of 5-6 different exercises, each one requiring you to complete 5 SETS of each. Between exercises take your time adjusting your weights or having a sip of water, there is no rush to start the next exercise. Obviously don't go and make a cup of tea and cool down, but don't get flustered unscrewing dumbbells or hurriedly moving your Swiss ball away (the rule of the '45 second break between SETS' applies only to the current exercise you are doing).

As mentioned in the previous chapter, we will be **TRAINING 3 DAYS IN A ROW AND THEN RESTING FOR 1 DAY** (then repeating this for the next 3 months!). For this reason, and to allow rest for the larger muscles, I designed 3 different workouts; one workout for each day of the three training days (and on each of these three days you target a different large muscle group). This breakdown is as follows:

DAY ONE: CORE, CHEST and ARMS

DAY TWO: CORE, BACK and ARMS

DAY THREE: CORE, SHOULDERS and ARMS

Before I now detail the specifics of each workout, I want to say that everyday we will be performing one variety of PRESS-UP and one variety of BICEP CURL. You may say this contradicts what I've just said about resting the different muscle groups, but the point is not training the muscle to *complete exhaustion* again, and by carrying out one SET of PRESS-UPS, for example, on the day after working the chest out to exhaustion will not put your body under undue stress.

Don't worry if you don't know what the names of the exercises are yet, the *Exercises* section features detailed, annotated images which describe each one.

There may also be instructions along the lines of 'ON BOTH SIDES' or 'FOR BOTH THE LEFT AND RIGHT SIDE.' These mean that the exercise has to be repeated for both your left and ride side of the body. Whatever the described body positioning for these exercises, reverse it for performing the exercise on the opposite side.

If there are 10 REPS of an exercise and there is an instruction 'FOR BOTH THE LEFT AND RIGHT SIDE' that means the 10 REPS have to be performed on both the left AND ride side; making a total of 20 REPS even though the exercise only states 10.

If the exercise is called 'ALTERNATING ARM…..' (followed by the name of an exercise) it means you perform one REP with one arm, and the next REP with the other arm, and so on, ALTERNATING YOUR ARMS until you have completed the required number of REPS.

THE 'BE RAD' WORKOUT PLANS

CORE WORKOUT [*PERFORM THIS SAME ROUTINE BEFORE EVERY WEIGHT WORKOUT*]
1 SET: 20 REPS: SWISS BALL SIT-UPS
2 SETS: 10 REPS: SWISS BALL OBLIQUE TWISTS: **BOTH LEFT AND RIGHT SIDE**
1 SET: 20 REPS: SWISS BALL OBLIQUE SIT-UPS: **BOTH LEFT AND RIGHT SIDE**
1 SET: 20 REPS: FACE-DOWN SWISS BALL LEG RAISES
1 SET: 20 REPS: INDIVIDUAL TWISTING LEG RAISES: **BOTH LEFT AND RIGHT SIDE**
1 SET: 20 REPS: ROLLING SWISS BALL ABDOMINAL PUSH
1 SET: 20 REPS: SWISS BALL WALL SQUATS

DAY ONE: CHEST and ARMS
5 SETS in PYRAMID SET STRUCTURE: 20, 18, 16, 14 then 12 REPS: PARALLEL GRIP PRESS-UPS
5 SETS: 16 REPS: LEGS RAISED LAYING FLIES
5 SETS: 12 REPS: CLOSE-GRIP PRESS-UPS
5 SETS: 8 REPS: PARALLEL GRIP TRICEP EXTENSION: **SUPERSET with: 8 REPS:** HORIZONTAL GRIP TRICEP EXTENSION
5 SETS: 20 REPS: ALTERNATING ARM HAMMER CURLS: **SUPERSET with: 8 reps:** ALTERNATING ARM BICEP CURLS
5 SETS in PYRAMID SET STRUCTURE: 20, 18, 16, 14 then 12 REPS: HORIZONTAL GRIP PRESS-UPS

DAY TWO: BACK and ARMS
5 SETS: 16 REPS: SINGLE ARM BENT OVER DUMBBELL ROW: **BOTH LEFT AND RIGHT SIDE**
5 SETS: 16 REPS: BENT OVER LATERAL RAISE
5 SETS: 20 REPS: ALTERNATING ARM BICEP CURLS: **SUPERSET with: 8 reps:** ALTERNATING ARM HAMMER CURLS
5 SETS: 12 REPS: CLOSE GRIP PRESS-UPS
5 SETS: 21 REPS: 21s

DAY THREE: SHOULDERS and ARMS
5 SETS: 14 REPS: ARNIE PRESS
5 SETS: 12 REPS: LATERAL RAISE
5 SETS: 30 REPS: ALTERNATING ARM FRONT DUMBBELL RAISE
5 SETS: 16 REPS: SEATED OVERHEAD TRICEP EXTENSION: **BOTH LEFT AND RIGHT ARM**
5 SETS: 20 REPS: ALTERNATING ARM HAMMER CURLS: **SUPERSET** with: 8 reps: ALTERNATING ARM BICEP CURLS
5 SETS in PYRAMID SET STRUCTURE: 20, 18, 16, 14 then 12 REPS: HORIZONTAL GRIP PRESS-UPS

11. THE EXERCISES

How I Keep My Legs Strong

Before I jump into explaining the exercises, I want to address the fact that I don't have a solely 'Leg Training Day' and apart from the SWISS BALL WALL SQUAT there are no exercises that seem to target the muscles in your legs. Due to the damage to my knees I spoke about earlier, I have to avoid overusing these joints and causing myself discomfort and risking further injury (especially with all the walking, swimming, working, travelling, exercising and socialising I already do). Here is how I keep the muscles in my legs strong (and you will to) without ever training them to exhaustion:

- All of the CORE EXERCISES involve using your whole body, including your LEGS, to position and balance yourself.
- For every SET with weights you do, you will be lifting the dumbbells off the floor and placing them back down again. Making sure you lift with the CORRECT FORM of **BENDING AT THE KNEES AND KEEPING YOUR BACK STRAIGHT** will mean that the muscles in you LEGS are doing the work to push all the weight of your upper body and the added weight of the dumbbells back upright. The same applies to placing the dumbbells back on the floor (during any one of the **'BE-RAD' WORKOUTS** you will be doing this about 30 times).
- Most of our weightlifting exercises will be performed standing up, so of course the muscles in your LEGS and CORE will be holding you, and that extra weight, in position for the entire time you are doing that exercise (for almost the whole WORKOUT then!).
- Walk rather than use transport (when this is a realistic option!) to get to work, do the shopping, meet friends, get across town, use stairs instead of a lift, etc. (I do **A LOT** of walking and think that

plays a big part in my overall fitness: I work a full time job that requires me to work on my feet the entire time, on my days off I walk 2 miles to town, walk around town for a couple of hours, then walk the same 2 miles back home, then walk another mile later to my local supermarket and then another mile home carrying my food shopping).

Hopefully from this you can see that the muscles in your legs *will* be worked while following the '**BE RAD' WORKOUT PLANS**.

If your knees aren't quite as discombobulated as yours truly, then by all means research LEG exercises you are able to perform. They are *big, powerful* muscles that burn *a lot* of fuel! You use them every day, they will help and assist you your entire life. Train them and look after them (and your joints as well!).

Stretching and Flexing

Our CORE workout serves as our main warm-up, but it is important to limber up and stretch your muscles before lifting heavy weights. The idea of stretching is very simple, you want to get your muscles ready for action and get blood pumping to anywhere that it is about to be needed. Flexing your muscles (though don't hold your breath or force blood to rush to your head) will also pump your muscles full of blood; flex between exercises and after you've finished lifting weights to maximise your results. Pictured here are the stretches and flexes I regularly perform before, during and after exercise to fill my muscles with that all-important blood. There are no rules on SETS or REPS for stretches, just perform a few (4-8) of each until you can feel your muscles 'waking-up.'

[Some of the images have been rotated to fit the page; you may need to turn the book horizontally to view the images in their intended orientation]

STRETCHES

CHEST PUSH

1. Lift your right elbow to shoulder height at your side, bend that arm 90 degrees and open your hand with the palm facing forward.
2. Press your left palm against your forward-facing right palm.
3. Apply resistance with your left arm and push forward against this resistance with your bent right arm until it is straight.
4. Return to original position and repeat.
5. Perform on your LEFT SIDE as well.

75

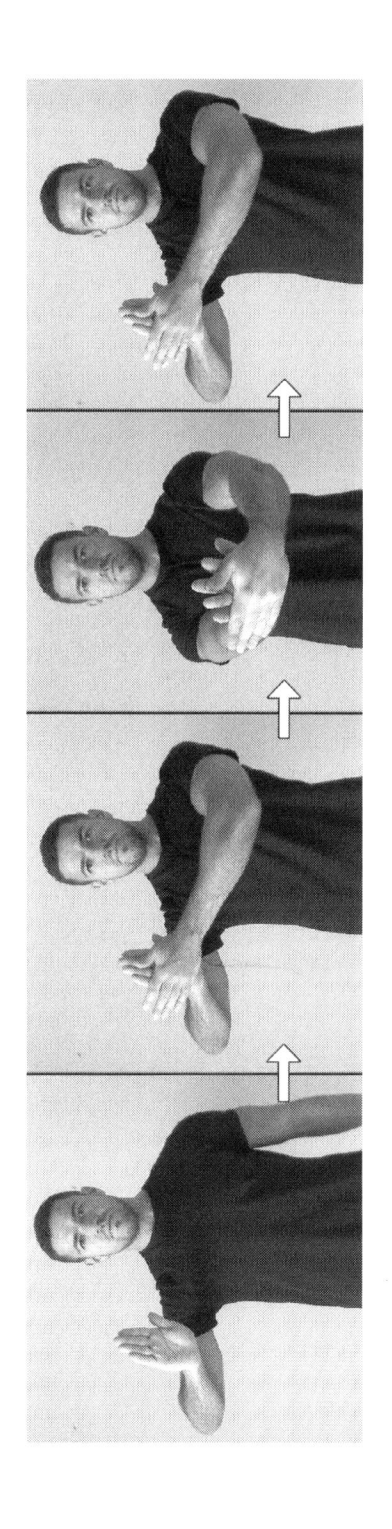

CHEST STRETCH

1. Stretch your right arm out straight to side and raised at shoulder height.
2. Place your open palm against the corner of a wall or surface.
3. Keeping your arm straight, twist your body until you can feel the muscles in that side of your CHEST stretch.
4. Perform on your LEFT SIDE as well.

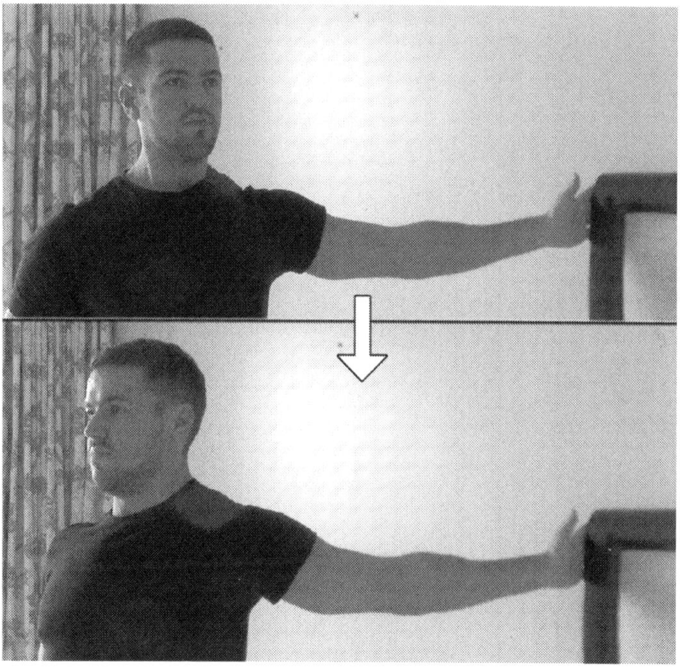

BICEP STRETCH

1. Starting with your right arm hanging at your side with your palm facing forward, place your left palm against the inside of your right wrist.
2. Apply resistance with your left arm and try to curl your right arm (as if you were performing a BICEP CURL).
3. Return to original position and repeat.
4. Perform on your LEFT SIDE as well.

79

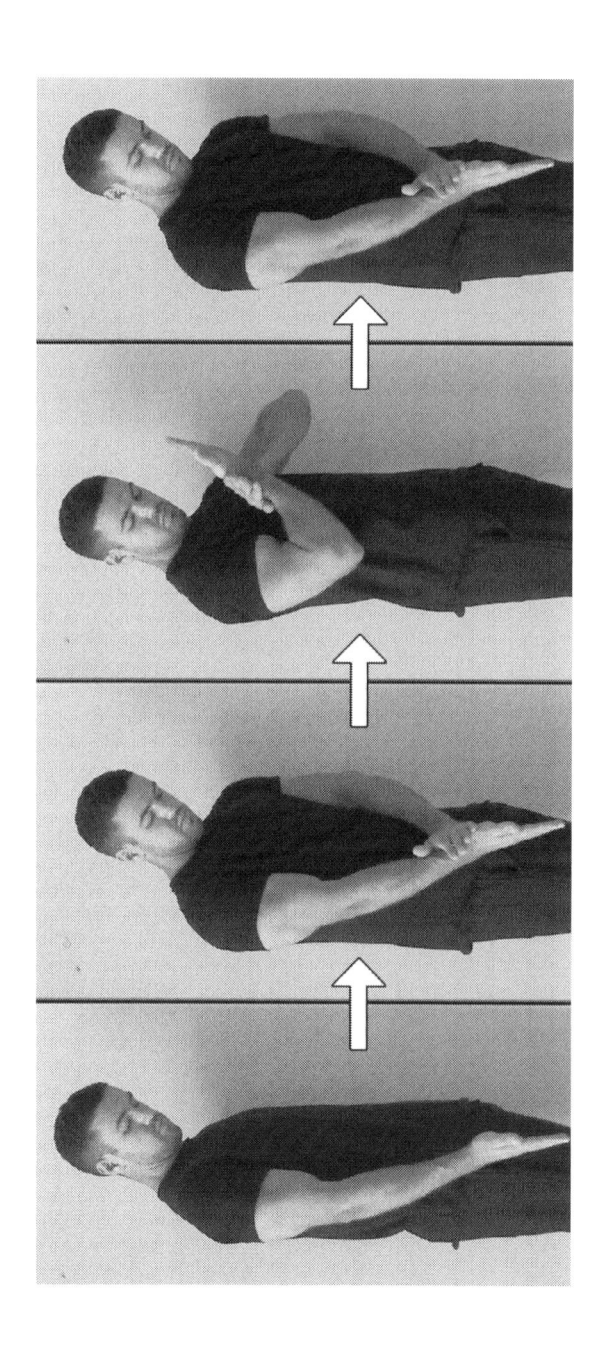

TRICEP STRETCH

1. Starting with your right arm bent in front of you, with your elbow close to your body and your right hand in front of your right shoulder, place your left palm against the bottom of your right hand.
2. Apply resistance with your left arm and push your right hand downwards against it.
3. Return to original position and repeat.
4. Perform on your LEFT SIDE as well.

81

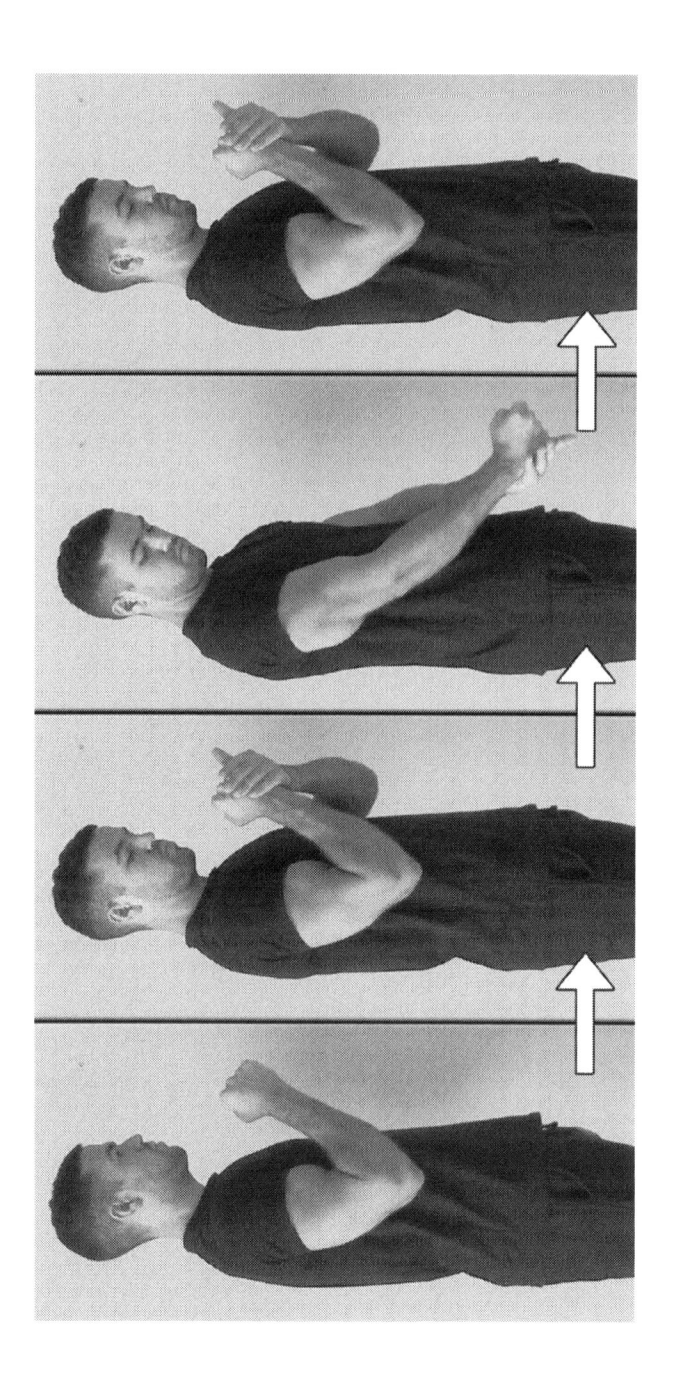

SHOULDER ROTATIONS

1. With your arms outstretched, slowly move them in complete circles around the side of your body (reaching as far back as you can).
2. Perform them rotating your arms forwards and also perform them rotating your arms backwards.

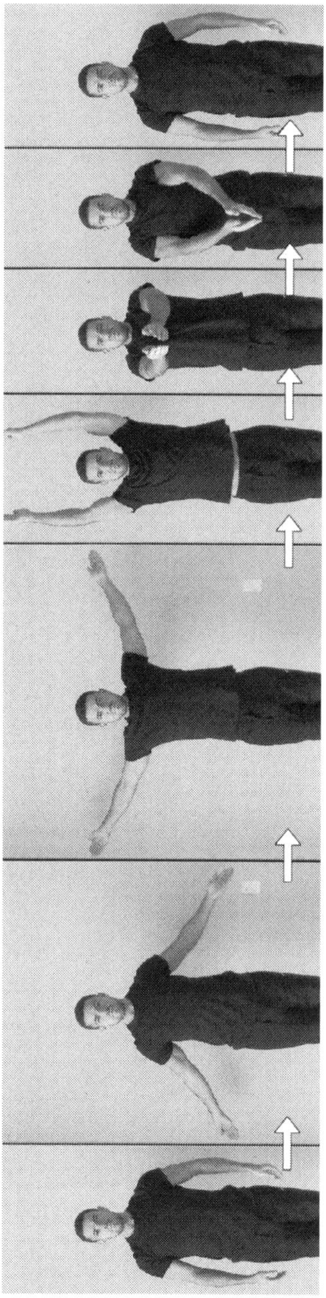

BENT OVER ROWING

1. Bend at the knees, keep your back straight and head up.
2. Starting with your arms hanging loosely towards the floor, pull both your elbows up towards your side.
3. Return your arms to their original position and repeat.

85

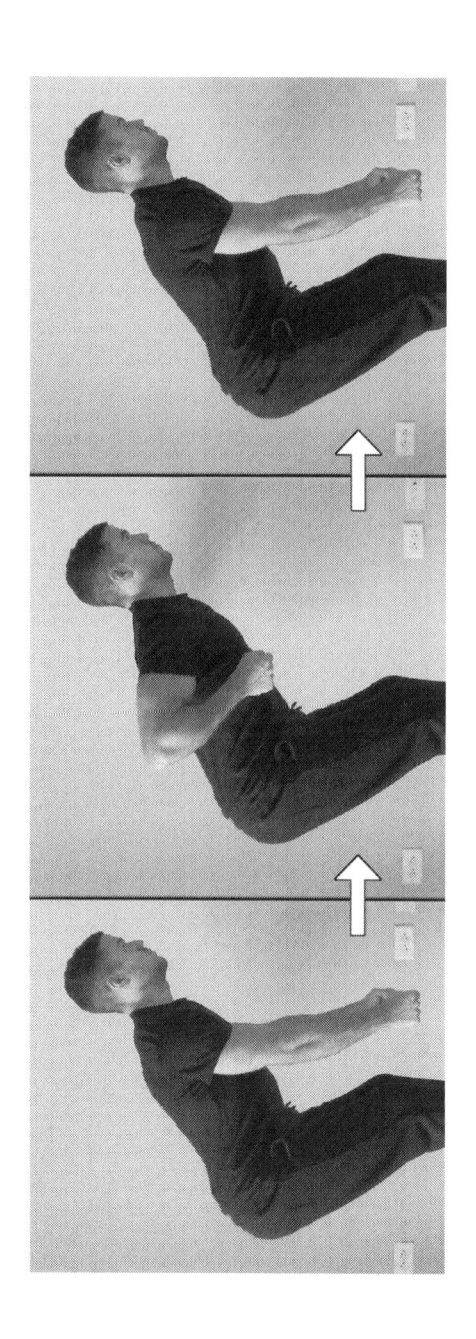

PUNCHING

1. Punch the air alternating between your left and right hands.

87

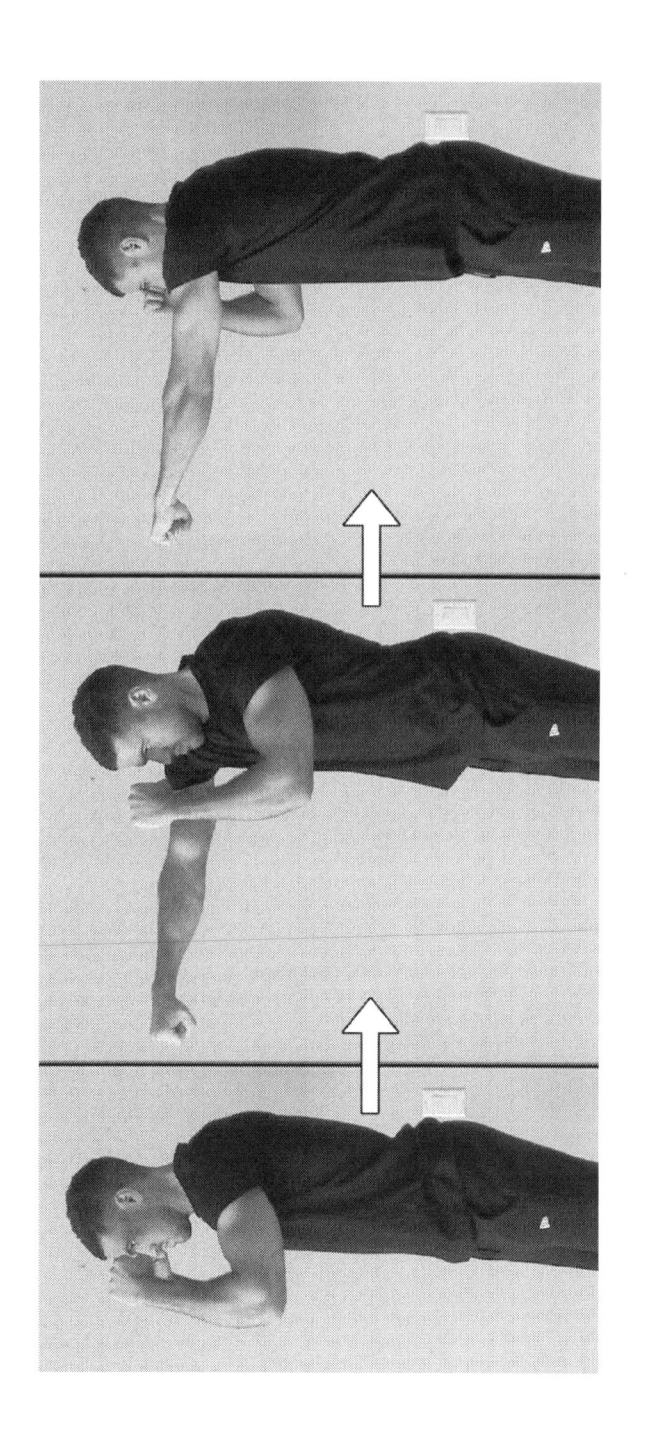

CORE WORKOUT EXERCISES

SWISS BALL SIT-UPS   :**1 SET: 20 REPS**

1. With your buttocks on one side of the SWISS BALL, lay horizontally with your legs bent at about a 90 degree angle. Your feet should be firmly flat on the floor. You can use your toes to anchor yourself to a wall in order to stabilise yourself.
2. With your hands either lightly resting on your thighs or against the side of your head and keeping your back straight, slowly raise your upper body while keeping your lower body perfectly still. DO NOT SIT UP ALL THE WAY. You should only raise yourself up to around 30 – 40 degrees. This range of motion targets the abdominal muscles in your stomach and won't over-involve the lower back (which sitting up all the way will).
3. Once at the peak of the SIT-UP, slowly lower your upper body back to its starting position, ready for the next **REP**.

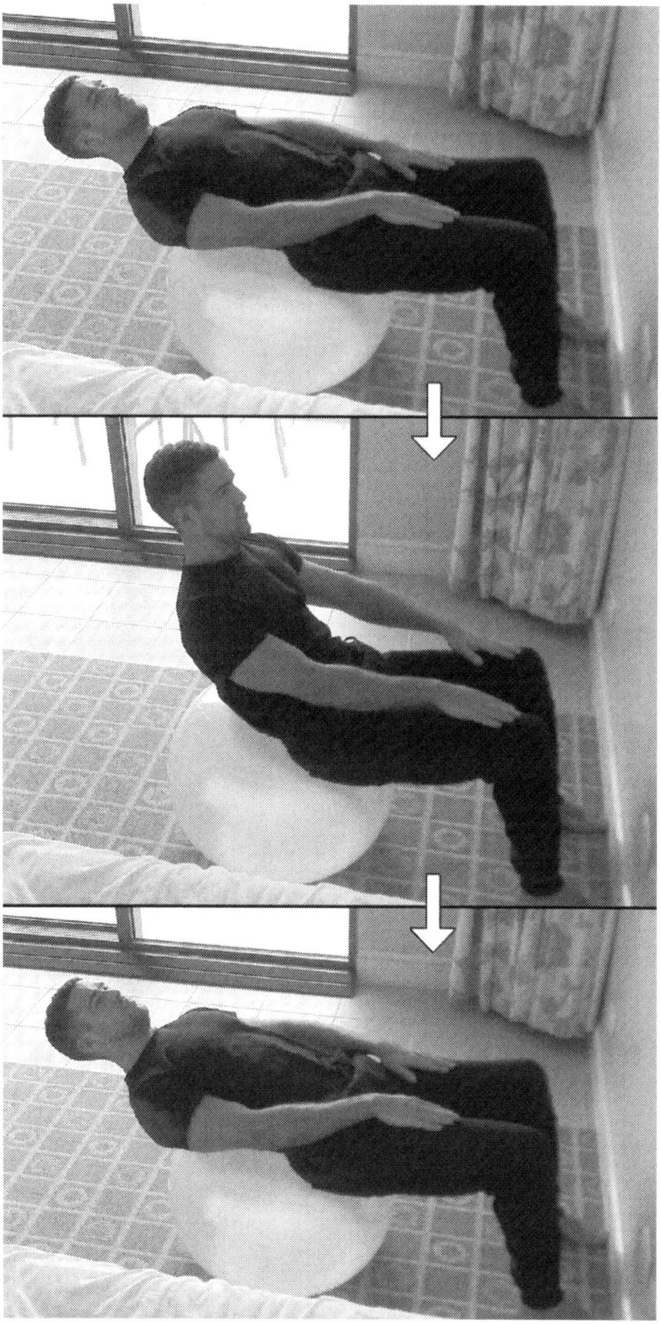

SWISS BALL OBLIQUE TWISTS :**2 SETS: 10 REPS (BOTH SIDES)**

1. With your buttocks on one side of the SWISS BALL, lay horizontally with your legs bent at about a 90 degree angle. Your feet should be firmly flat on the floor. You can use your toes to anchor yourself to a wall in order to stabilise yourself.
2. Place your right hand on your left shoulder and loosely place your left hand on your left thigh.
3. Keeping your back straight, slowly raise your upper body and with your left hand reach forward and across to try and touch the outside of your right knee. Depending on how flexible you are will determine if you can actually touch the outside of your knee. It doesn't matter if you can't touch the outside of your right knee, what is important is that you are sitting-up and reaching across your body at the same time.
4. Though you shouldn't be aiming to sit all the way up, you may raise your upper body slightly higher than you did with the regular SWISS BALL SIT-UP.
5. Once you have reached the peak of your SITTING-UP and reaching towards your right knee, slowly lower your upper body and left hand back to their starting positions, ready for the next **REP**.
6. After the first **10 REPS** touching your right knee with your left hand, swap sides (place your left hand on your right shoulder and your right hand on your right thigh – you will be reaching towards your left knee with that right hand) and perform another **10 REPS**. Have a 45 second break then perform another full **SET**.

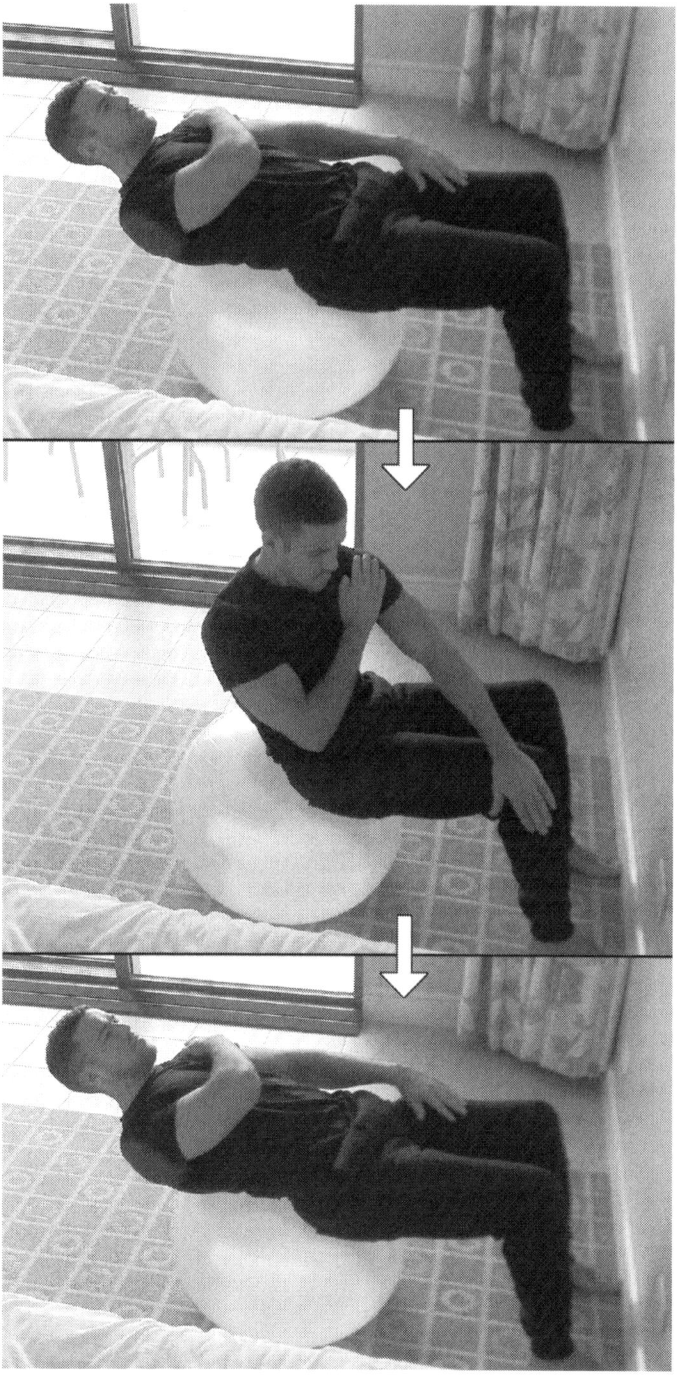

SWISS BALL OBLIQUE SIT-UPS :**1 SET: 20 REPS (BOTH SIDES)**

1. For this exercise you need to position the SWISS BALL close enough to a wall so that you can brace your feet against it.
2. Rest the outside of your left thigh against one side of SWISS BALL, bend your left leg at the knee, push it out in front of you and wedge your foot into the edge between the floor and the wall. Stretch your right leg out behind you and wedge your right foot into the edge between the floor and the wall. The position of your legs should almost resemble a 'lunging' position – though resting diagonally with your left thigh on the SWISS BALL.
3. At this point your body should be facing in the left direction. While leaving your crotch facing in this left direction, turn your shoulders until you are facing the wall (you can stretch your arms out in front of you to maintain your balance). This is the starting position for this exercise.
4. Keeping your lower body in the same position, raise your upper body towards the wall as far as you can. You should feel the muscles in the side of your mid-section working hard.
5. Once you have reached the peak of your SIT-UP, slowly lower your upper body back to its starting position, ready for the next **REP**.
6. After **20 REPS** on this side, swap to the other side and perform **20 REPS**.
7. NOTE: DUE TO THE TWISTED POSITION OF YOUR BODY INVOLVED IN THIS EXERCISE, MAKE SURE YOU KEEP AN EYE ON YOUR FORM, PERFORM EACH REP SLOWLY AND IN A CONTROLLED MANNER.

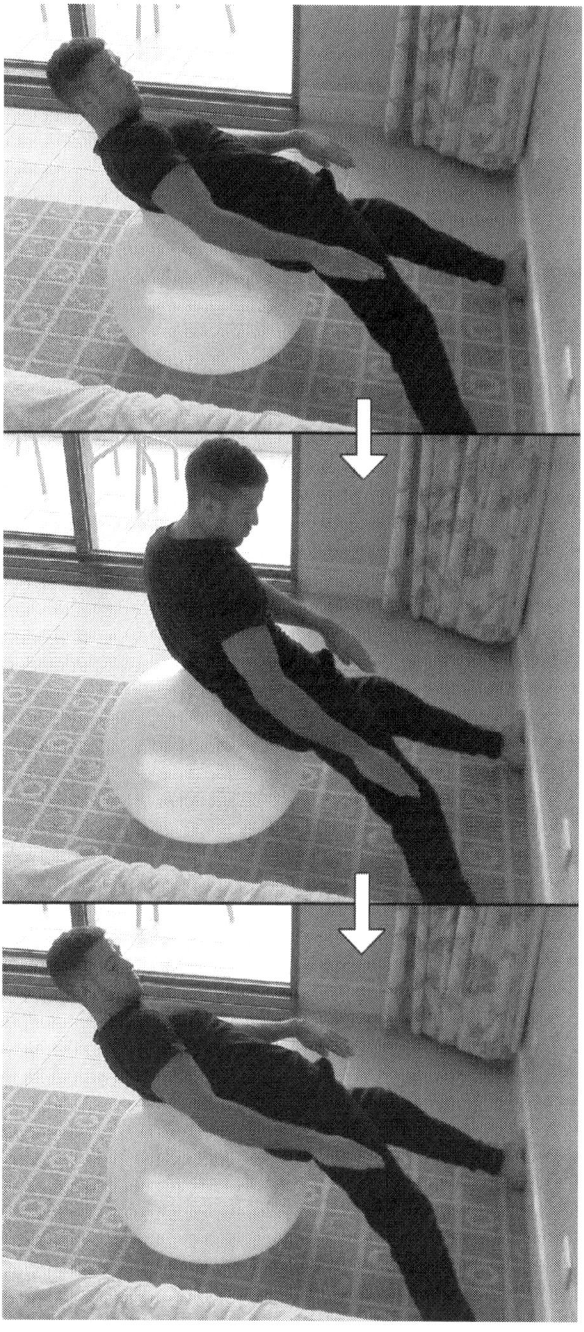

FACE-DOWN SWISS BALL LEG RAISES   :**1 SET: 20 REPS**

1. Lay face-down on top of the SWISS BALL, with the SWISS BALL positioned underneath your crotch. Lift your chin up and keep your back straight. Place the palms of your hands flat against the floor, keep your legs out straight with your knees and heels together. This is the starting position for this exercise
2. Keep your upper body and the SWISS BALL in the same positions. Then with your legs still straight, raise both of your heels at the same time as far as you can.
3. You should feel the muscles in your lower back working hard.
4. Once you have lifted your heels as high as you can, slowly lower them back to the starting position, ready for the next **REP**.

97

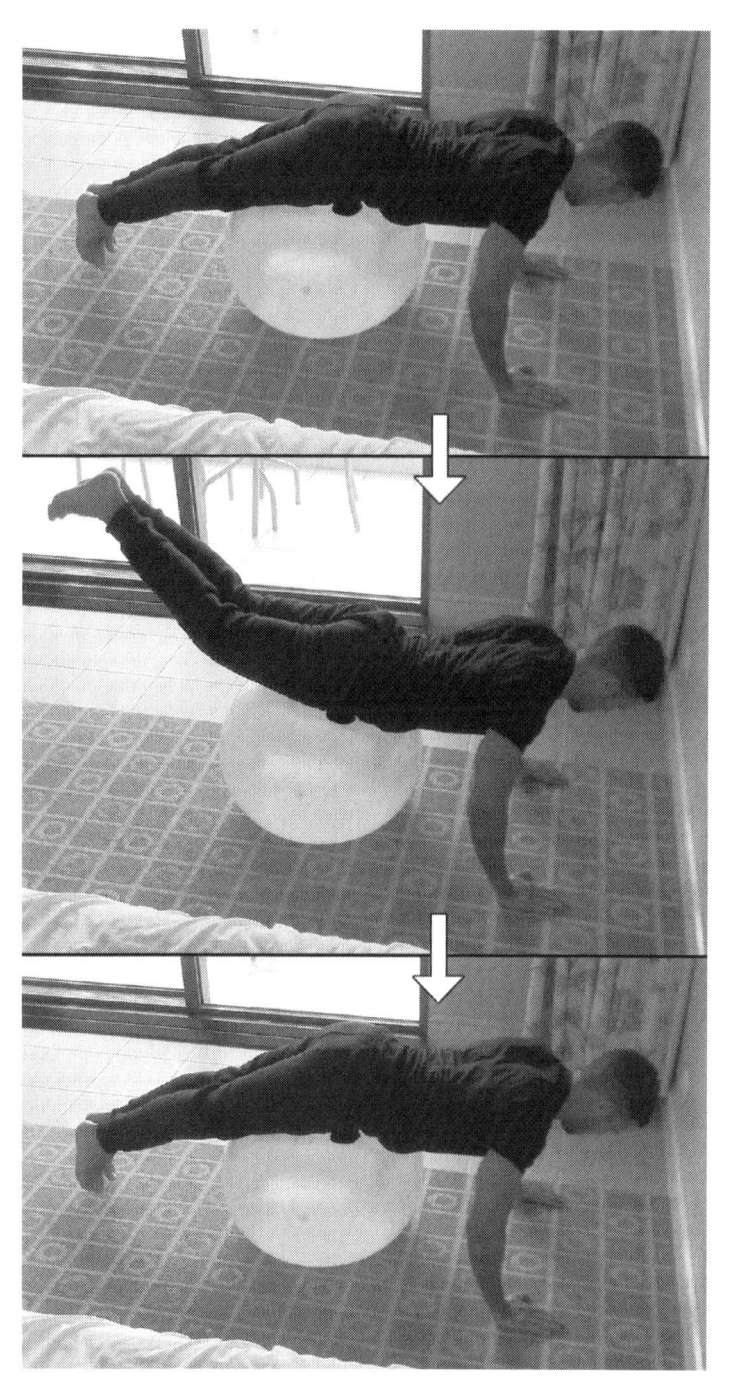

INDIVIDUAL TWISTING LEG RAISES   :**1 SET: 20 REPS (BOTH SIDES)**

1. Lay on the ground on your left side, with your body completely straight. Place your left arm under your head for support and your right arm on the floor in front of you for balance. While keeping your legs together at the knees, twist your right leg so your toes point towards the ground. This is the starting position for this exercise.
2. Keep the rest of your body in the same position and slowly raise your right leg, keeping it held straight at the knee. AS YOU RAISE YOUR RIGHT LEG, ROTATE IT AT THE HIP SO THAT YOUR FOOT GOES FROM POINTING DOWNWARDS TO POINTING TOWARDS THE CEILING.
3. Once you have raised your leg as high as you can, slowly lower it back to its starting position, ready for the next **REP**. MAKE SURE YOU ROTATE YOUR LEG AT THE HIP ON ITS WAY BACK DOWN, SO YOUR FOOT TURNS FROM POINTING AT THE CEILING BACK TO POINTING TOWARDS THE GROUND.
4. After **20 REPS** on this side, swap to laying on your right side and perform **20 REPS** with your left leg.

99

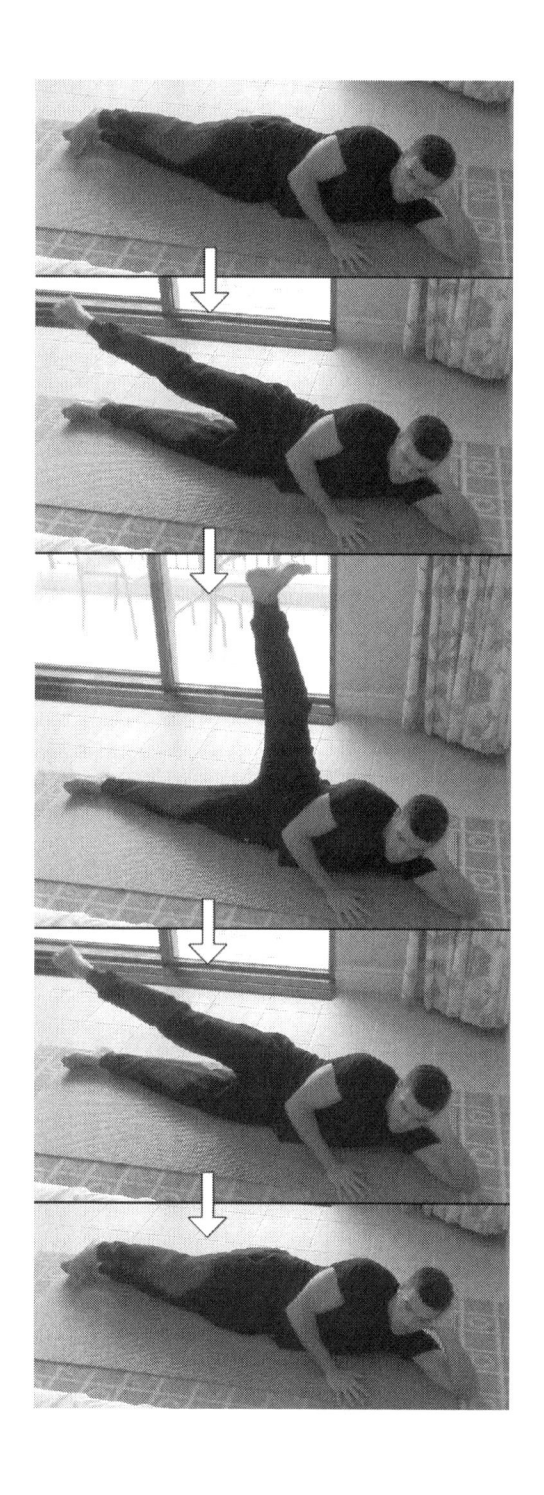

ROLLING SWISS BALL ABDONIMAL PUSH   :**1 SET: 20 REPS**

1. Lay flat on the ground looking up, with the back of your ankles resting on the SWISS BALL. You should have your feet about 6 inches apart. Your buttocks should not be in contact with the floor. Stretch your arms out slightly to the side of your body, spread your fingers on each hand and press your fingertips against the floor. Your forearm, elbow and upper arms SHOULD NOT BE IN CONTACT WITH THE FLOOR. Your fingertips are only there to assist with balancing (if you are resting your bodyweight via your arms touching the floor, you ruin the performance of this exercise). This is the starting position for this exercise.
2. Drag the SWISS BALL towards you using your heels until your legs are bent towards your chest and your feet are flat on the surface of the SWISS BALL.
3. With your feet flat on the SWISS BALL holding it in position, push with your legs and push your crotch into the air. When your thighs, mid-section and stomach align, you have reached the peak of this exercise.
4. Slowly lower your crotch back to where it just was, so your knees are bent towards your chest again.
5. Now roll the SWISS BALL away from you using the soles of your feet, roll it until it is once again resting under your ankles and your legs are straight. You should have returned to your starting position and are ready for the next **REP**.

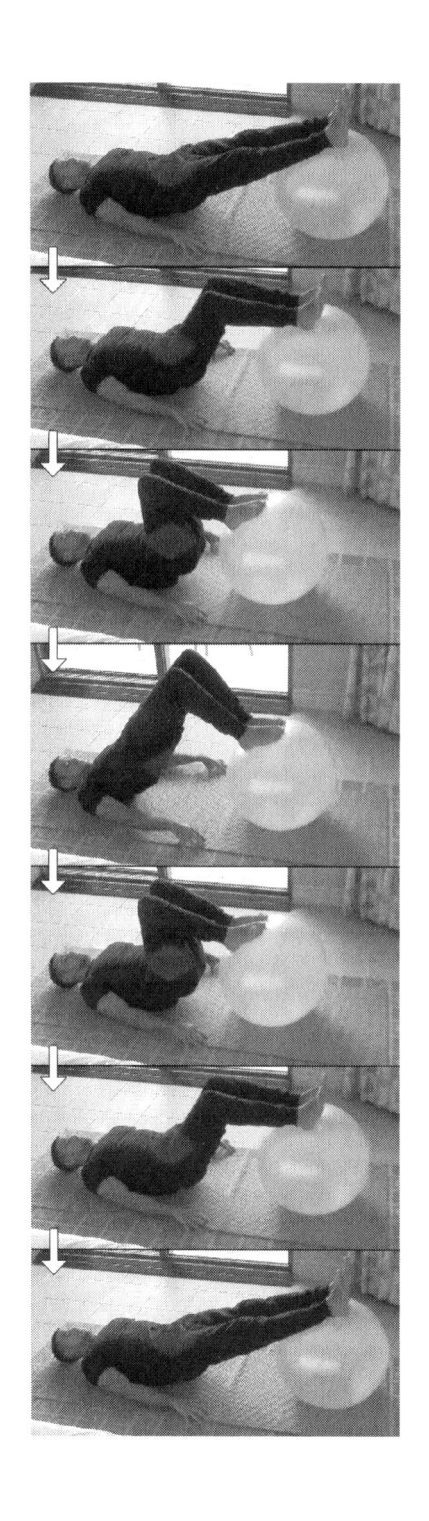

SWISS BALL WALL SQUATS :**1 SET: 20 REPS**

1. Place the SWISS BALL between you and a wall; it should be positioned at your lower back. Place your feet in front of you and shoulder width apart. Very slightly bend your knees to prepare your muscles and joints, DON'T LOCK YOUR KNEES STRAIGHT. How far in front you place your feet depends on the length of your legs, when you squat in a moment you want your knees to just reach over your toes; so at the bottom of this exercise your legs are bent at about a 90 degree angle. You may place your arms crossed over your chest, hold them straight out in front of you or let them hang at your side. This is the starting position for this exercise.
2. Holding the SWISS BALL against the wall with your lower back, slowly bend your legs and lower your body, as though you were going to sit down. The SWISS BALL should roll up your back as your body lowers.
3. Lower yourself until your knees are bent close to a 90 degree angle. (I have to be very careful with this exercise and even when I do it my knees grate, lock and pop, it can be very unpleasant for me and I only do it to keep my leg muscles alive! Know your limits and lower yourself as far as you are comfortable with and without comprising the controlled form of the exercise.)
4. Once at the lowest point, push up with your legs and raise your body. Still holding the SWISS BALL between yourself and the wall, it should now be rolling back to its original position at your lower back.
5. Once you have returned to the starting position you are ready for the next **REP**.

[IF YOU HAVE PERFECTLY HEALTHY KNEES AND LEGS YOU CAN ADD SOME WEIGHT TO THIS EXERCISE. WITH YOUR ARMS HANGING AT YOUR SIDE, ALL YOU HAVE TO DO IS HOLD A DUMBBELL OF THE SAME WEIGHT IN EACH HAND, AND KEEP HOLD OF THAT WEIGHT AT YOUR SIDE WHILE YOU SQUAT UP AND DOWN.]

103

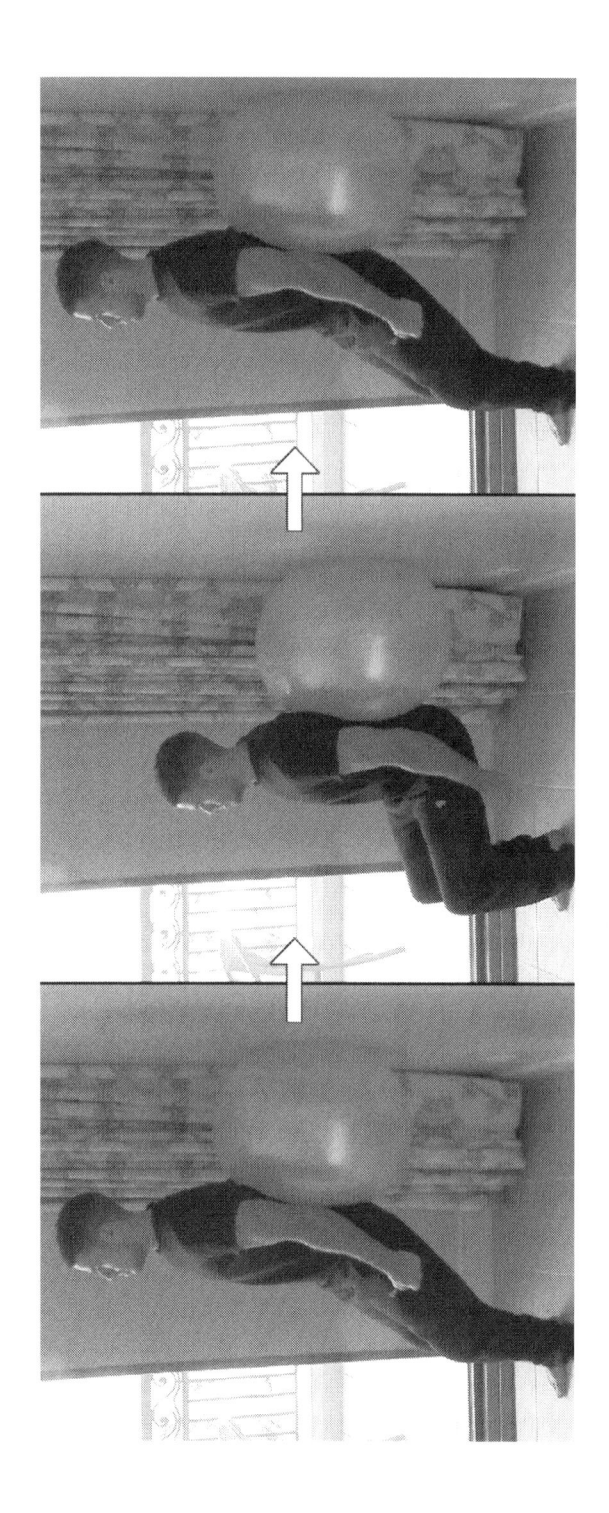

DAY ONE: CHEST and ARMS EXERCISES

PARALLEL GRIP PRESS-UPS :**5 SETS in PYRAMID SET STRUCTURE: 20, 18, 16, 14 then 12 REPS**

1. Place your PRESS-UP handles on the floor running parallel to your body, and in line with your chest. They should be wider apart than your shoulders. (Wide enough apart so that when you lower yourself your arms bend through a perfect 90 degree angle during the PRESS-UP movement.)
2. Grip the handles, hold your bodyweight up (your arms should have a slight bend and not be 'locked' at the elbows) and position your legs behind you. Your feet and legs should be together and your entire body (legs and back) should be completely straight. Lift your chin up slightly and look forward. This is the 'top' of the PRESS-UP and the starting position for this exercise.
3. Slowly lower your body towards the floor keeping your feet together and your legs and back straight. Lower yourself until your crotch is about to touch the floor. Your arms will bend through the 90 degree angle and your chest should be in between your PRESS-UP handles. If you have kept your body perfectly straight your chest, chin and face won't be anywhere near touching the floor before your crotch. DON'T PUSH YOUR CROTCH FORWARD / DOWN IN AN ATTEMPT TO TOUCH THE FLOOR, **KEEP YOUR BODY STRAIGHT!**
4. Once you have reached the 'bottom' of the PRESS-UP, slowly push your body back to its starting position ready for the next **REP**. Make sure you keep your body straight and legs and feet together on your way back up.
5. Remember, the **PYRAMID SET** structure means the number of **REPS** in your **5 SETS** is **20 REPS, 18 REPS, 16 REPS, 14 REPS and then 12 REPS**.

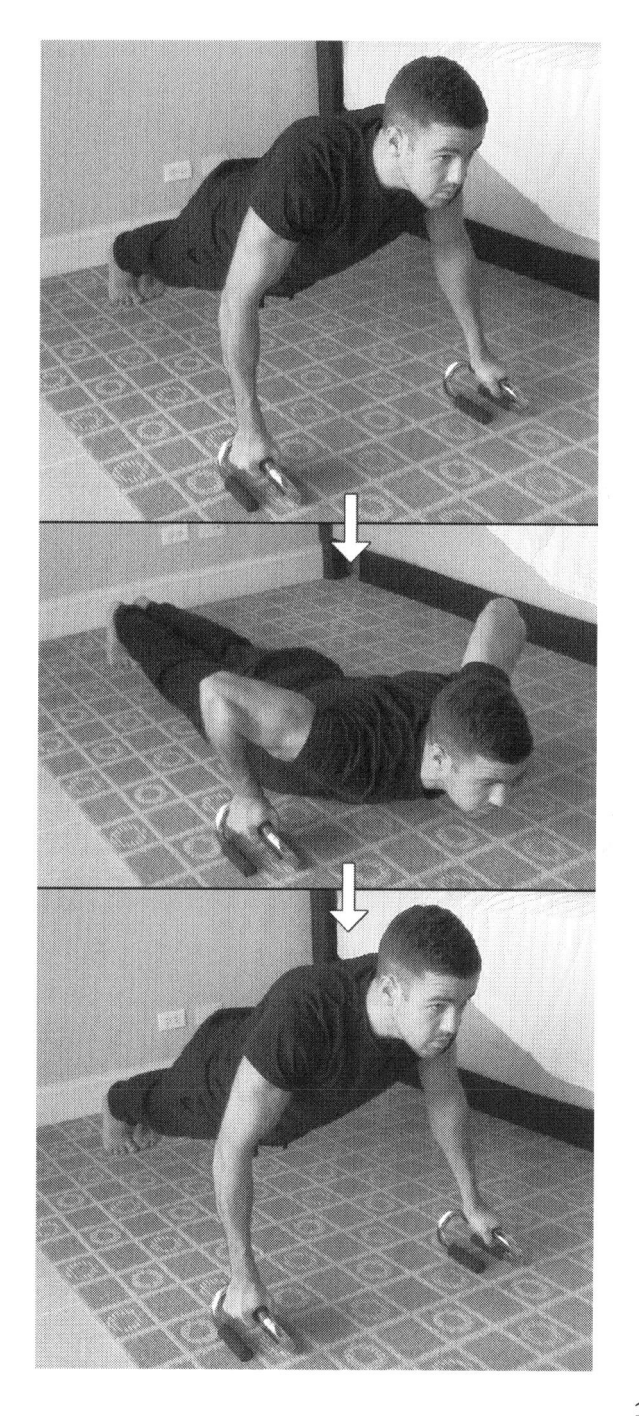

LEGS RAISED LAYING FLIES :**5 SETS: 16 REPS**

1. Lay on your back looking at the ceiling with your legs raised at a 90 degree angle to your body. Stretch your arms out to your sides and grip the DUMBBELLS with your palms facing towards the ceiling. This is the starting position for this exercise.
2. While keeping your legs at that 90 degree angle and your arms straight (without locking your elbows), slowly bring the DUMBBELLS together so they meet in the centre above your chest.
3. Keep your legs at 90 degrees, your arms straight and slowly lower the DUMBBELLS back to their starting position ready for the next **REP**. (BUT CONTROL THE WEIGHT AND TRY NOT TO LET THE DUMMBELLS TOUCH THE FLOOR! This would deactivate the muscles you're trying to exhaust after every **REP**. This might seem tricky at first, and even I sometimes end up letting them touch the floor, BUT *REALLY* TRY NOT TO LET THIS HAPPEN.)

109

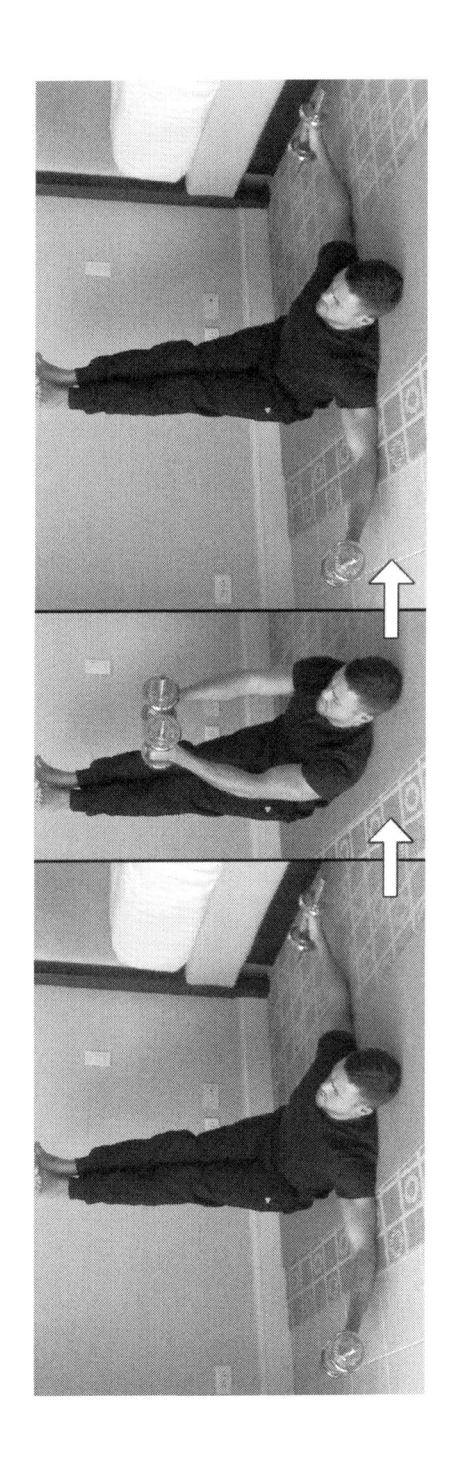

CLOSE-GRIP PRESS-UPS :5 SETS: 12 REPS

1. Place your PRESS-UP handles as close together as you can get them and horizontally in line with each other. With your arms outstretched (without locking your elbows) the handles should be positioned below your chest. Keep your feet together and your legs and your back straight. Lift your chin up and look forward. This is the starting position for this exercise.
2. Slowly lower your body towards the floor, keeping your legs together and your body straight. You should lower yourself until your chest just touches the top of your hands.
3. Push your body back to its starting position ready for the next **REP**.

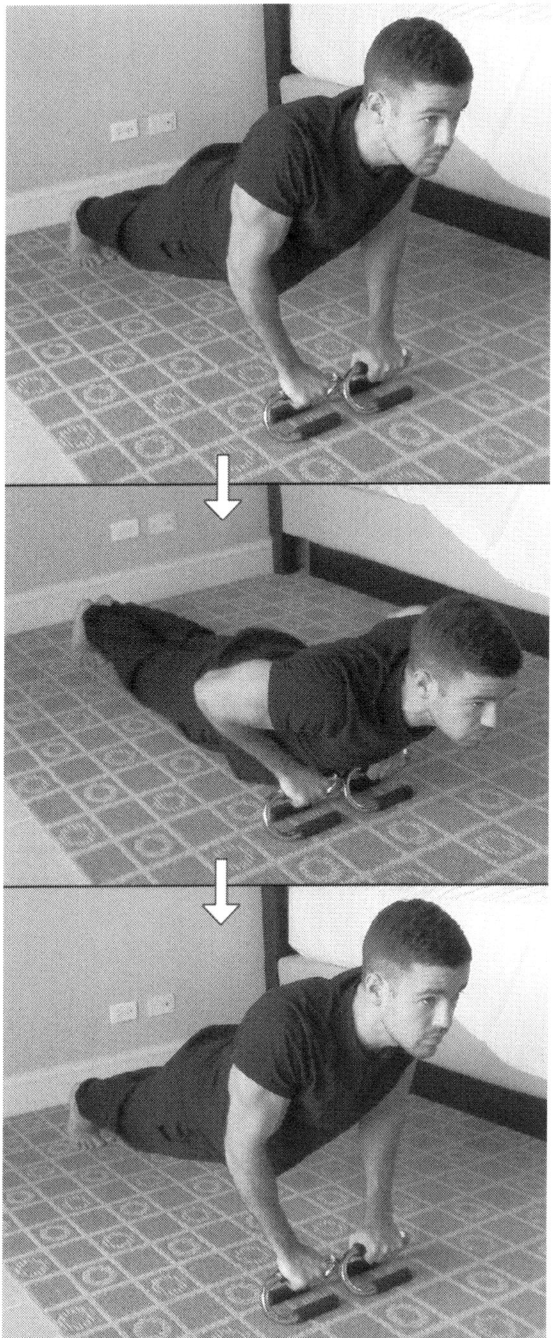

PARALLEL GRIP TRICEP EXTENSION :5 SETS: 8 REPS
SUPERSET WITH
HORIZONTAL GRIP TRICEP EXTENSION :5 SETS: 8 REPS

1. With your feet close together, bend your knees slightly, push your bum out and lower your upper body until it is almost horizontal, keeping your back straight and your head up. PAY CLOSE ATTENTION TO MAINTAINING YOUR POSTURE FOR THIS EXERCISE DUE TO THE EXTRA WORKLOAD ON YOUR LOWER BACK.
2. With your arms bent grip a DUMBBELL in each hand. For the PARALLEL GRIP TRICEP EXTENSION you want your palms facing inwards towards each other; so the bars in the DUMBBELLS are pointing in the same direction that you are looking (forward). This is the starting position for this exercise.
3. Keep your body in that same position, including your shoulders and upper arms. The only parts of your body that move during this exercise are your lower arms. Pay extra attention to making sure your elbows don't move. Now extend both your hands out backwards until your bent arms become straight.
4. In a controlled manner, bend your arms again and bring the weights back to their original position ready for the next **REP**. (Again making sure you keep your body, especially your upper arms, in the same position).
5. After **8 REPS** holding the DUMBBELLS parallel to your body, twist your hands outwards 90 degrees (while keeping the rest of your body in the same position); the DUMBBELLS would have rotated and are now horizontally in line with each other and at 90 degrees to the imaginary line down which you are facing. Your palms should be facing forwards. Now you will perform **8 REPS** of HORIZONTAL GRIP TRICEP EXTENSIONS without having had a 45 second break (THIS IS A **SUPER SET**).
6. Extend both of your hands out backwards until your bent arms become straight. (Watch out your elbows don't move!)

7. Slowly bend your arms again and bring the weights back to their original position ready for the next **REP**.
8. After your **8th REP** of the HORIZONTAL GRIP TRICEP EXTENSION, you have completed **1 SET**. Have your 45 second break now and prepare to start with the **8 REPS** of PARALLEL GRIP TRICEP EXTENSIONS again.

PARALLEL GRIP
TRICEP EXTENSION

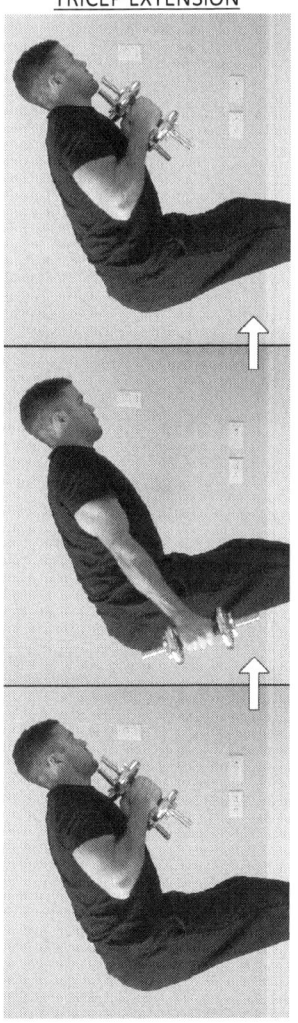

HORIZONTAL GRIP
TRICEP EXTENSION

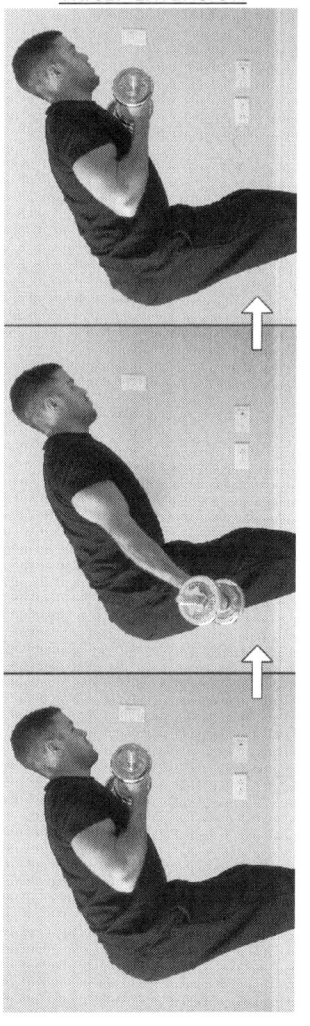

ALTERNATING ARM HAMMER CURLS :**5 SETS: 20 REPS**
SUPERSET WITH
ALTERNATING ARM BICEP CURLS :**5 SETS: 8 REPS**

1. Stand with your feet shoulder width apart and grip a DUMBBELL in each hand with your arms down at your side. Your palms should be facing inwards towards your thighs.
2. Without moving your elbow, bend your right arm and bring the DUMBBELL towards your chest, keeping your hand and wrist in the same position so the DUMBBELL doesn't rotate at all. It should seem as though you are doing a 'skiing' motion with the DUMBBELL. This is an ALTERNATING ARM exercise so don't do anything with your left arm yet.
3. Once you have bent your right arm as much as you can and have brought the DUMBBELL up to your chest, slowly lower your right arm and return the DUMBBELL to its original position at your side. **THAT IS 1 REP.**
4. As soon as your right arm is back where it started, bend your left arm in the same manner and bring that DUMBBELL up to your chest. Keeping your elbow where it is and not rotating the DUMBBELL at all.
5. Once you have fully bent your left arm and have that DUMBBELL at your chest, slowly lower your left arm and return the DUMBBELL to its original position at your side. **THAT IS YOUR 2ND REP.**
6. As soon as your left arm is back where it started, perform another **REP** with your right arm. Continue this process until you have completed **20 REPS**. Which would work out at having performed **10 REPS** with each arm.
7. Without having a 45 second break, rotate your hands 90 degrees outwards so the bars of the DUMBBELLS are horizontally in line with each other. Your palms should be facing forwards. This is where we **SUPER SET** the ALTERNATING ARM BICEP CURLS.
8. Bend your right arm in the same controlled manner and bring the DUMBBELL to your chest; without moving your elbow or rotating the DUMBBELL as it moves.
9. Lower your right arm and return the DUMBBELL to its original position at your side. **THAT IS 1 REP.**

10. As before, bend your left arm now and bring that DUMBBELL to your chest.
11. Once you have brought that DUMBBELL fully to your chest lower it slowly back to its original position. **THAT IS YOUR 2ND REP.**
12. As soon as your left arm is back where it started, perform another **REP** with your right arm. Continue this process until your have completed **8 REPS**. Which would work out at having performed **4 REPS** with each arm.
13. Now have your 45 second break and prepare to start with the **20 REPS** of ALTERNATING ARM HAMMER CURLS again.

ALTERNATING ARM
HAMMER CURLS

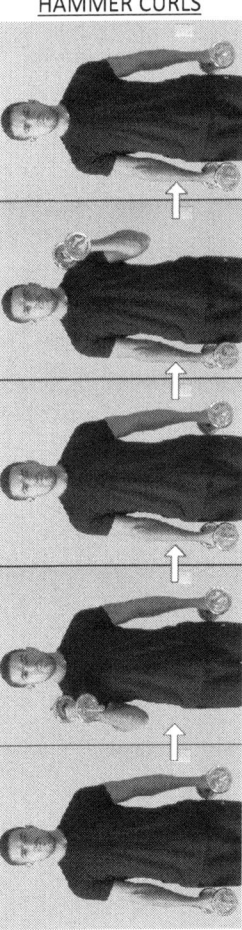

ALTERNATING ARM
BICEP CURLS

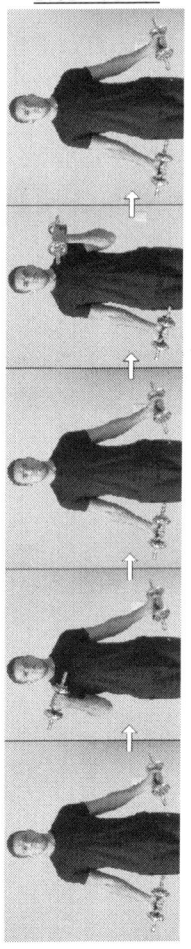

HORIZONTAL GRIP PRESS-UPS : 5 SETS in PYRAMID SET STRUCTURE: 20, 18, 16, 14 then 12 REPS

1. Place your PRESS-UP handles on the floor so they are horizontally in line with each other, they should also be in line with your chest. They should be wider apart than your shoulders. (Wide enough apart so that when you lower yourself your arms bend through a perfect 90 degree angle during the PRESS-UP movement.)
2. Grip the handles, hold your bodyweight up (your arms should have a slight bend and not be 'locked' at the elbows) and position your legs behind you. Your feet and legs should be together and your entire body (legs and back) should be completely straight. Lift your chin up slightly and look forward. This is the 'top' of the PRESS-UP and the starting position for this exercise.
3. Slowly lower your body towards the floor keeping your feet together and your legs and back straight. Lower yourself until your crotch is about to touch the floor. Your arms will bend through the 90 degree angle and your chest should be in between your PRESS-UP handles. If you have kept your body perfectly straight, your chest, chin and face won't be anywhere near touching the floor before your crotch. DON'T PUSH YOUR CROTCH FORWARD / DOWN IN AN ATTEMPT TO TOUCH THE FLOOR, **KEEP YOUR BODY STRAIGHT!**
4. Once you have reached the 'bottom' of the PRESS-UP, slowly push your body back to its starting position ready for the next **REP**. Make sure you keep your body straight and legs and feet together on your way back up.
5. Remember, the **PYRAMID SET** structure means the number of **REPS** in your **5 SETS** is **20 REPS, 18 REPS, 16 REPS, 14 REPS and then 12 REPS**.

117

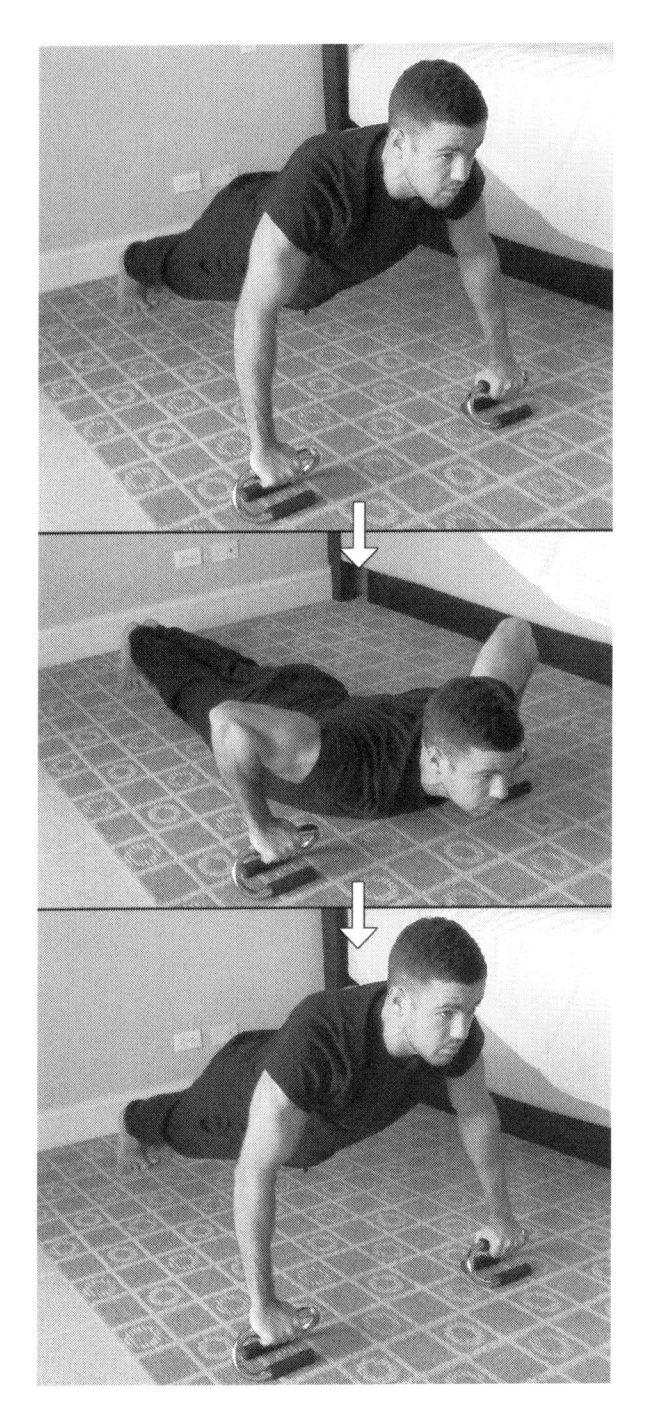

DAY TWO: BACK and ARMS EXERCISES

SINGLE ARM BENT OVER DUMBBELL ROW :5 SETS: 16 REPS: BOTH LEFT AND RIGHT SIDE

1. Place your left foot out in front of you and your right leg out behind you, bend forward on your left leg; you should be in a 'lunging' position. Rest your left forearm across your left thigh for support, keep your back straight, head up and hold the DUMBBELL with your right hand; your right arm should be hanging straight below your mid-section (the DUMBBELL shouldn't be touching the floor). This is the starting position for this exercise.
2. Keeping your body in that starting position and your back straight, pull the DUMBBELL towards your mid-section. Make sure you are using the muscles in your back, not lifting your shoulder up or twisting your body to trick yourself into thinking the DUMBBELL has been raised. ONLY YOUR ARM SHOULD BE MOVING, not your shoulder, waist or anything else.
3. Once the DUMBBELL has reached your mid-section, slowly lower it back to its original position ready for the next **REP**.
4. After **16 REPS** on your right side, don't have a 45 second break, swap straight to your left side and perform **16 REPS** on that side. Then have your 45 second break, before starting your next **SET** on the right side again.

121

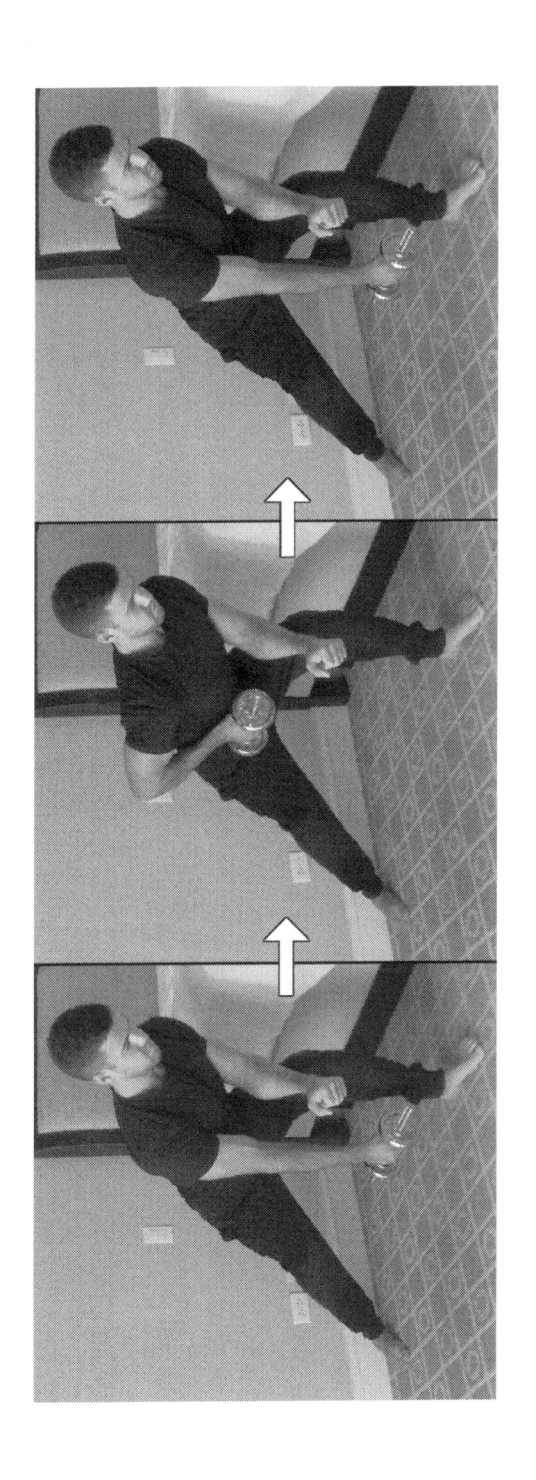

BENT OVER LATERAL RAISE :5 SETS: 16 REPS

1. With your feet together, slightly bend your knees and bend at the waist so your upper body is positioned horizontally. Lift your head up and keep your back straight. Hold a DUMBBELL in each hand, with your palms facing inwards towards each other. Your arms should be hanging straight down towards the floor; the DUMBBELLS shouldn't touch the floor. This is the starting position for this exercise.
2. Keeping your body in that starting position and your arms straight (BUT NOT LOCKED AT THE ELBOW) lift both DUMBBELLS outwards simultaneously until they are at the same height as your shoulders.
3. Once you have lifted the DUMBBELLS to this height, slowly lower them back to their starting position with your arms still straight and using that same sweeping motion. You are then ready to perform the next **REP**.

*[IT IS VERY IMPORTANT WITH THIS EXERCISE TO KEEP YOUR ARMS STRAIGHT, NOT TO THROW YOUR BODY INTO THE MOVEMENT AND TO CONTROL THE DUMBBELLS AS YOU RAISE THEM **AND** AS YOU LOWER THEM. YOU ARE TRYING TO TARGET THE BACK OF YOUR SHOULDERS (REAR DELTOIDS) NOT YOUR ARMS, YOUR LOWER BACK OR ANYTHING ELSE. YOU MAY END UP USING A MUCH LIGHTER WEIGHT FOR THIS EXERCISE THAN YOU EXPECTED TO.]*

123

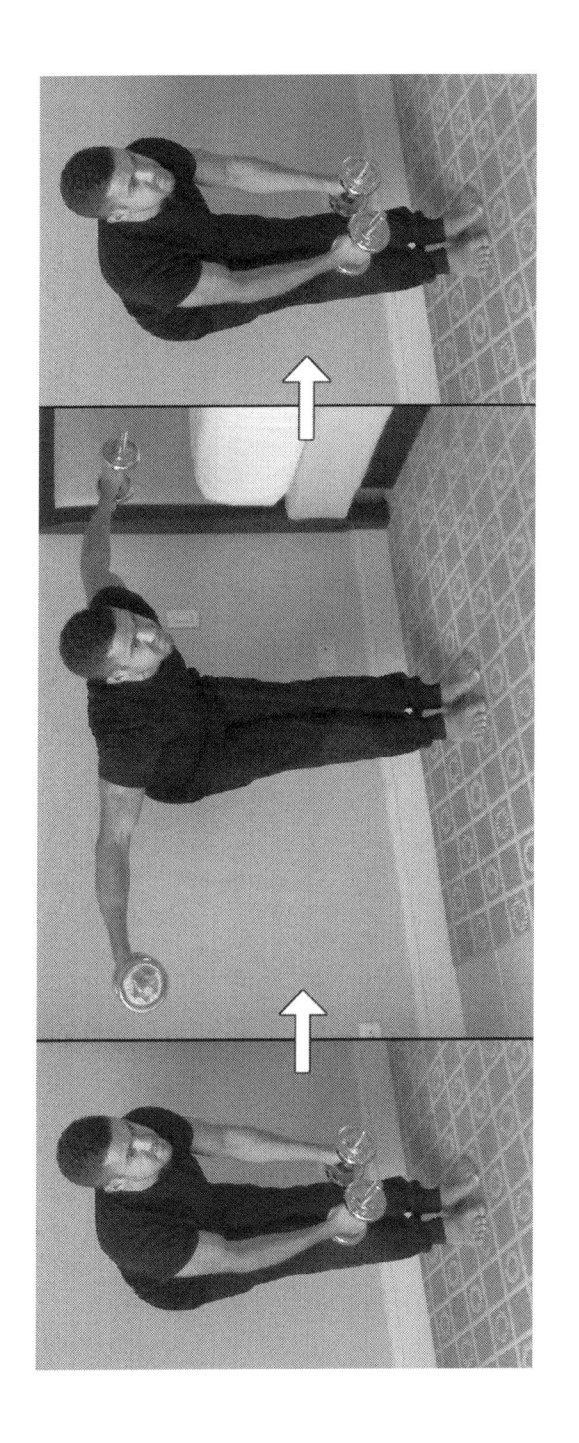

ALTERNATING ARM BICEP CURLS :**5 SETS: 20 REPS**
SUPERSET WITH
ALTERNATING ARM HAMMER CURLS :**5 SETS: 8 REPS**

1. Stand with your feet shoulder width apart and grip a DUMBBELL in each hand with your arms down at your side. Your palms should be facing forwards.
2. Without moving your elbow, bend your right arm and bring the DUMBBELL towards your chest, keeping your hand and wrist in the same position so the DUMBBELL doesn't rotate at all. This is an ALTERNATING ARM exercise so don't do anything with your left arm yet.
3. Once you have bent your right arm as much as you can and have brought the DUMBBELL up to your chest, slowly lower your right arm and return the DUMBBELL to its original position at your side. **THAT IS 1 REP.**
4. As soon as your right arm is back where it started, bend your left arm in the same manner and bring that DUMBBELL up to your chest. Keeping your elbow where it is and not rotating the DUMBBELL at all.
5. Once you have fully bent your left arm and have that DUMBBELL at your chest, slowly lower your left arm and return the DUMBBELL to its original position at your side. **THAT IS YOUR 2ND REP.**
6. As soon as your left arm is back where it started, perform another **REP** with your right arm. Continue this process until you have completed **20 REPS**. Which would work out at having performed **10 REPS** with each arm.
7. Without having a 45 second break, rotate your hands 90 degrees inwards so the bars of the DUMBBELLS are pointing forward and running parallel to each other. Your palms should be facing inwards towards your thighs. This is where we **SUPER SET** the ALTERNATING ARM HAMMER CURLS.
8. Bend your right arm in the same controlled manner and bring the DUMBBELL to your chest; without moving your elbow or rotating the DUMBBELL as it moves. It should seem as though you are doing a 'skiing' motion with the DUMBBELL.
9. Lower your right arm and return the DUMBBELL to its

original position at your side. **THAT IS 1 REP.**
10. As before, bend your left arm now and bring that DUMBBELL to your chest.
11. Once you have brought that DUMBBELL fully to your chest lower it slowly back to its original position. **THAT IS YOUR 2ND REP.**
12. As soon as your left arm is back where it started, perform another **REP** with your right arm. Continue this process until your have completed **8 REPS**. Which would work out at having performed **4 REPS** with each arm.
13. Now have your 45 second break and prepare to start with the **20 REPS** of ALTERNATING ARM BICEP CURLS again.

ALTERNATING ARM BICEP CURLS

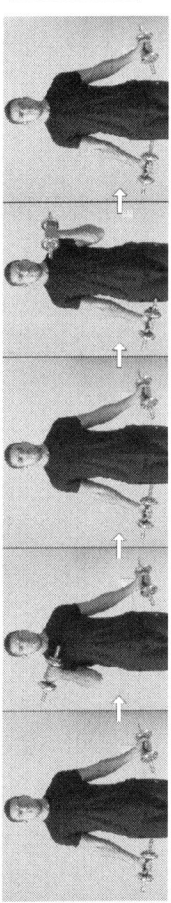

ALTERNATING ARM HAMMER CURLS

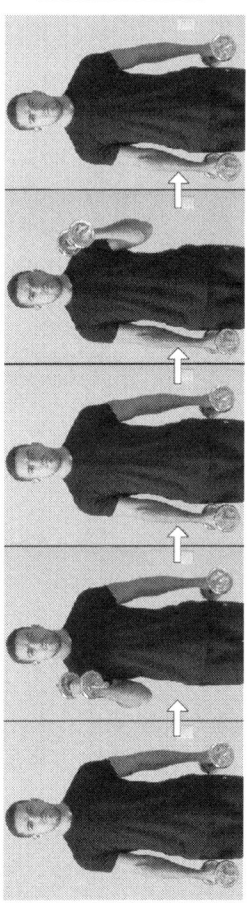

CLOSE-GRIP PRESS-UPS   :**5 SETS: 12 REPS**

1. Place your PRESS-UP handles as close together as you can get them and horizontally in line with each other. With your arms outstretched (without locking your elbows) the handles should be positioned below your chest. Keep your feet together and your legs and your back straight. Lift your chin up and look forward. This is the starting position for this exercise.
2. Slowly lower your body towards the floor, keeping your legs together and your body straight. You should lower yourself until your chest just touches the top of your hands.
3. Push your body back to its starting position ready for the next **REP**.

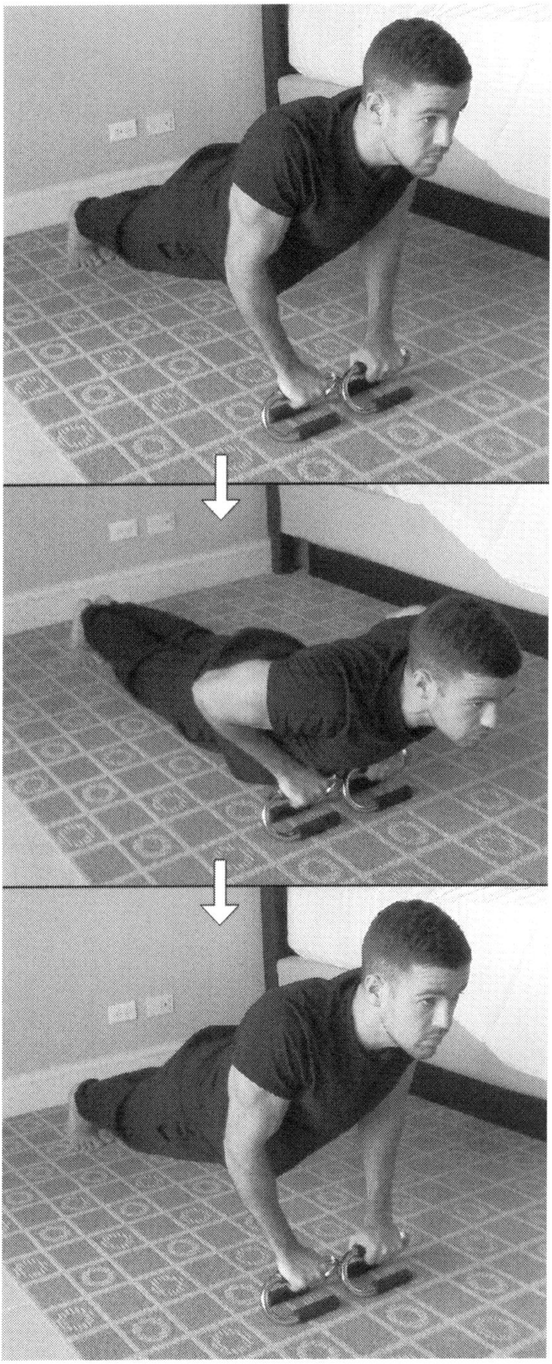

21s : 5 SETS: 21 REPS

'21s' are a BICEP CURLING EXERCISE that will fully stretch and workout EVERY part of your biceps. It will truly exhaust your arms performing this at the end of the workout.

1. Stand with your feet shoulder width apart and grip a DUMBBELL in each hand with your arms down at your side. Your palms should be facing forwards and the bars of the DUMBBELLS should be horizontally in line with each other. This is the starting position for this exercise.
2. Without moving your elbows, bend both your left and right arms at the same time, as though you were going to perform a traditional BICEP CURL, **BUT STOP THE MOVEMENT HALFWAY THROUGH, SO YOUR ARMS ARE BENT AT 90 DEGREES**. Controlling the weight, slowly lower the DUMBBELLS back to their starting position. That is **1 REP**.
3. Perform another **6 REPS** of BICEP CURLS **STOPPING THE DUMBBELLS AT 90 DEGREES (HALFWAY THROUGH THE MOVEMENT)**.
4. Once this first **7 REPS** have been completed and without having a 45 second break, bring the DUMBBELLS up to your chest; to what would be the final position of a FULL BICEP CURL. For the next **7 REPS** you will be lowering the DUMBBELLS from this position at your chest **DOWN TOWARDS THE HALFWAY POINT OF A FULL BICEP CURL**. That same halfway point you have just been stopping the DUMBBELLS at, only this time you are lowering the weight there from above, as opposed to lifting it there from below. Perform **7 REPS** lowering both DUMBBELLS to this halfway point simultaneously, and then slowly curling the DUMBBELLS back to the peak of the BICEP CURL at chest height.
5. Once you have completed these **7 REPS** lower the DUMBBELLS back to your side. Without having a 45 second break you are now going to perform **7 REPS** of FULL BICEP CURLS. Your palms should still be facing forward and the bars of the DUMBBELLS should still be horizontally in line with each other.

6. Curl both DUMBBELLS simultaneously, still without moving your elbows, all the way up to your chest for **7 REPS**.
7. Once you have completed these **7 REPS** you have completed **1 SET** of 21s. Now have your 45 second break in preparation for the next **SET**.

<u>21s: REPS 1-7</u>

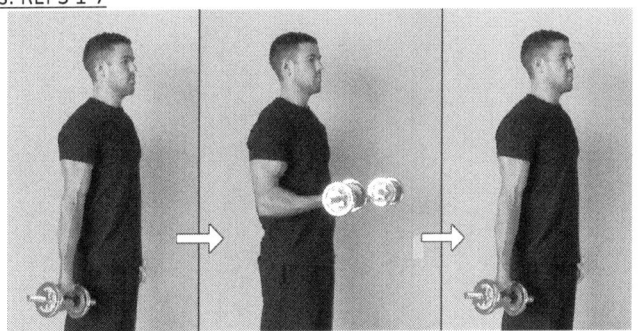

<u>21s: REPS 8-14</u>

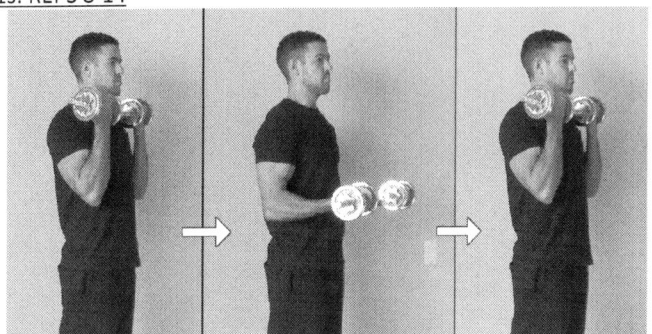

<u>21s: REPS 15-21</u>

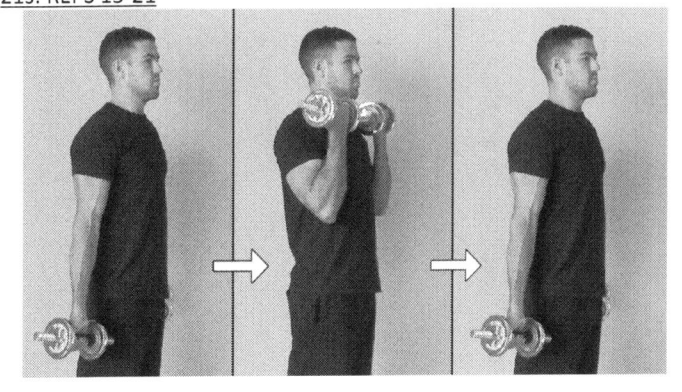

DAY THREE: SHOULDERS and ARMS EXERCISES

ARNIE PRESS : 5 SETS: 14 REPS

1. Stand upright with your feet shoulder width apart. Hold a DUMBBELL in each hand, with your arms completely bent and the DUMBBELLS in front of your chest. Your palms should be facing inwards, towards your chest, and the bars of the DUMBBELLS should be horizontally in line with each other. This is the starting position for this exercise.
2. Move both of your arms up and outwards at the same time, rotating your wrists outwards so your palms begin to turn forwards. Follow this motion until your elbows are at shoulder height, with a 90 degree bend in your arms at the elbow and your palms are completely facing forward; the bars of the DUMBBELLS should have moved through a 180 degree twist and be horizontally in line with each other again.
3. From here press the DUMBBELLS upwards towards the ceiling, until your arms are almost completely straight and the DUMBBELLS are almost touching.
4. To return to your starting position, simply complete the same movement in reverse. Controlling the weight, slowly lower your arms so your elbows are once again at shoulder height with a 90 degree bend at the elbow; your palms should be facing forward.
5. Now lower your arms inwards and twist your wrists inwards at the same time, rotating the DUMBBELLS. Your elbows should move down and towards your body and the DUMMBELLS should end up back where they started; in front of your chest with your palms facing inwards towards your chest. That is **1 REP**.
6. Perform another **13 REPS** and then have your 45 second break, in preparation for the next **SET**.

ARNIE PRESS:
LIFTING WEIGHT

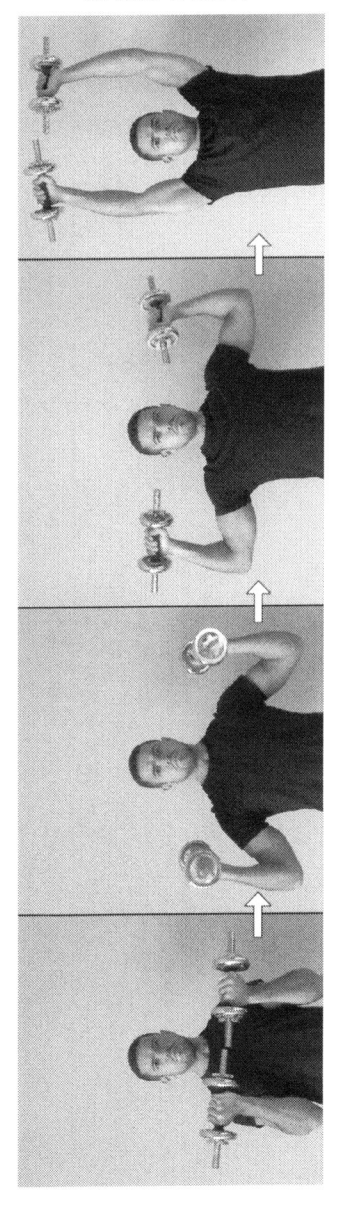

ARNIE PRESS:
LOWERING WEIGHT

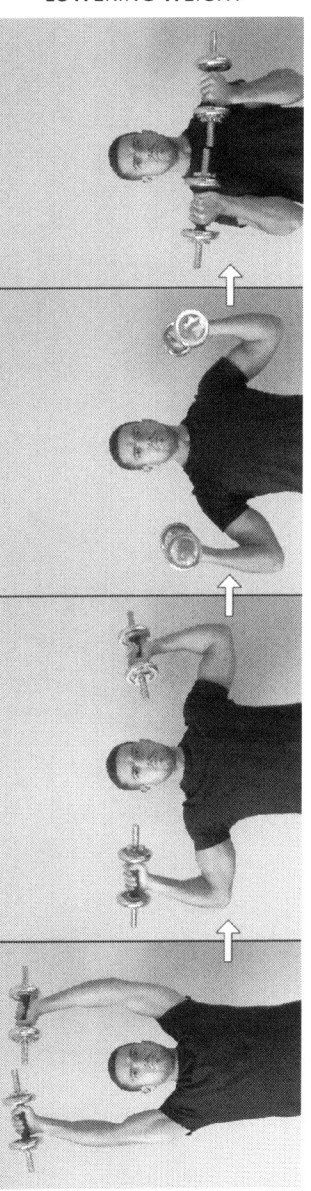

LATERAL RAISE :5 SETS: 12 REPS

1. Stand with your feet close together and grip a DUMBBELL in each hand with your arms down at your side. Your palms should be facing inward towards your thighs. This is the starting position for this exercise.
2. Keeping your back straight, head up and arms straight (but not locked at the elbow) lift both DUMBBELLS to shoulder height at the same time. There should be a 90 degree angle between your arms and your body.
3. Control the weight and while keeping your arms straight, slowly lower the DUMBBELLS back to their original positions at your sides, ready for the next **REP**.

135

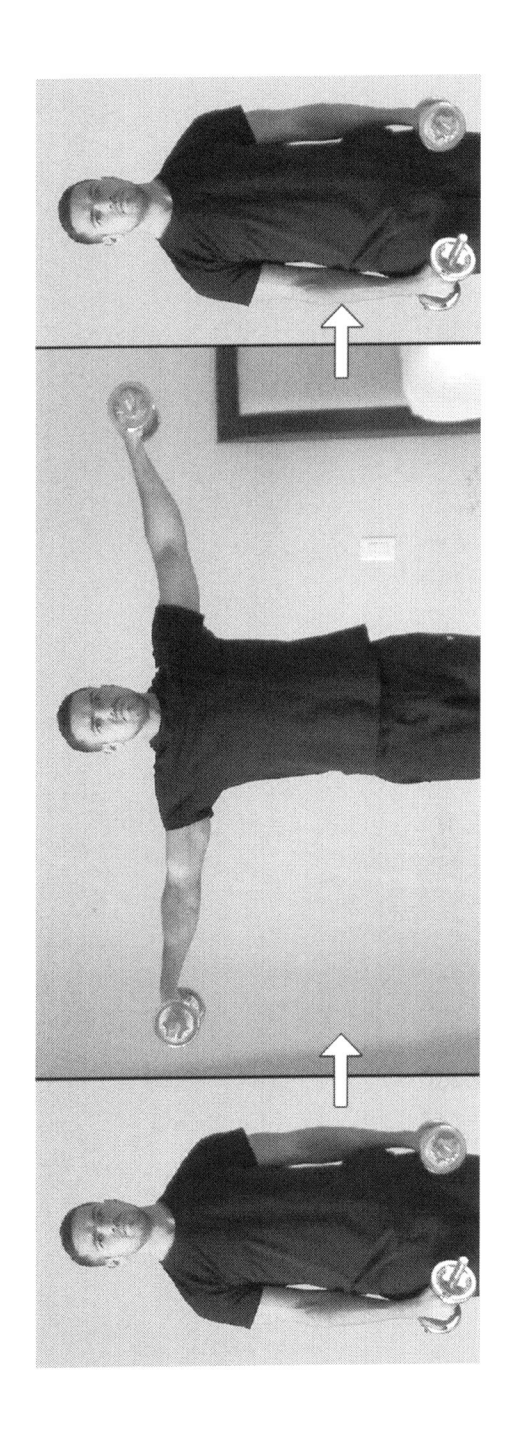

ALTERNATING ARM FRONT DUMBBELL RAISE :5 SETS: 30 REPS

1. Stand upright with your feet close together. Hold a DUMBBELL in each hand in front of your thighs. Your palms should be facing towards your body and the bars of the DUMBBELLS should be horizontally in line with each other. This is the starting position for this exercise.
2. Leave your left arm where it is (holding a DUMBBELL in front of your left thigh) and while keeping your right arm straight (but not locked at the elbow) lift the DUMBBELL in your right hand up, past your chest, past your face until your arm is pointing in the air and the DUMBBELL is well above head height.
3. Controlling the weight and while keeping your right arm straight, slowly lower the DUMBBELL back to its original position to complete the **1ST REP**.
4. Now lift the DUMBBELL in your left hand in exactly the same manner, all the way up until your arm is in the air and the DUMBBELL is above head height.
5. Controlling the weight and while keeping your left arm straight, slowly lower the DUMBBELL back to its original position to complete the **2ND REP**.
6. Perform another **REP** with your right arm, then left, and so and so forth until you have performed **15 REPS** with both arms (**30 REPS** in total). Then have your 45 second break in preparation for the next **SET**.

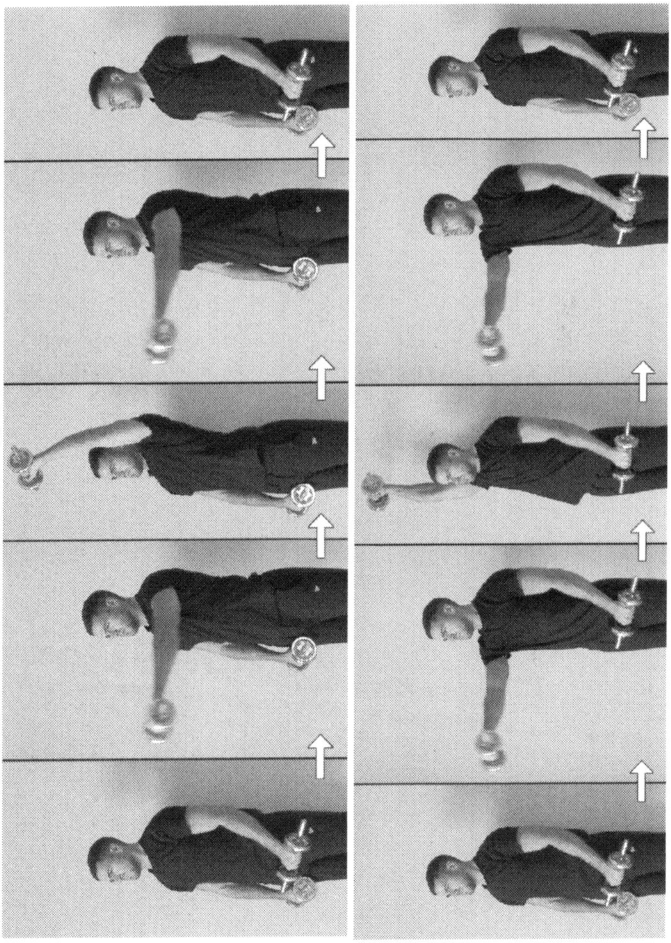

SEATED OVERHEAD TRICEP EXTENSION :5 SETS: 16 REPS: BOTH LEFT AND RIGHT ARM

1. Sit on a chair or the edge of a bed with your chest up and your back straight.
2. Hold a **DUMBBELL** in your right hand just above your head with your elbow bent. Place your left hand at the top of the right side of your chest for support. This is the starting position for this exercise.
3. Extend your right arm at the elbow and lift the **DUMBBELL** until your arm is straight. Your body, shoulder and upper arm should not move during this exercise. You are targeting your **TRICEPS** so only your lower arm extending the **DUMBBELL** should be moving.
4. Once your arm is completely extended, slowly lower the **DUMBBELL** back to its original position ready for the next **REP**.
5. Perform another **15 REPS** with your right arm and then without having a 45 second break swap sides.
6. Perform **16 REPS** with you left arm to complete the **1ST SET**. Now have your 45 second break in preparation for the next **SET**.

FORM AND CONTROL IN THIS EXERCISE ARE VITAL TO PREVENT INJURY! IF YOU OVERLOAD YOURSELF, THROW THE WEIGHT AROUND OR PERFORM THIS EXERCISE HASTILY THEN THAT VERY HARD, VERY METAL DUMBBELL MAY COLLIDE WITH YOUR VERY HUMAN SKULL!

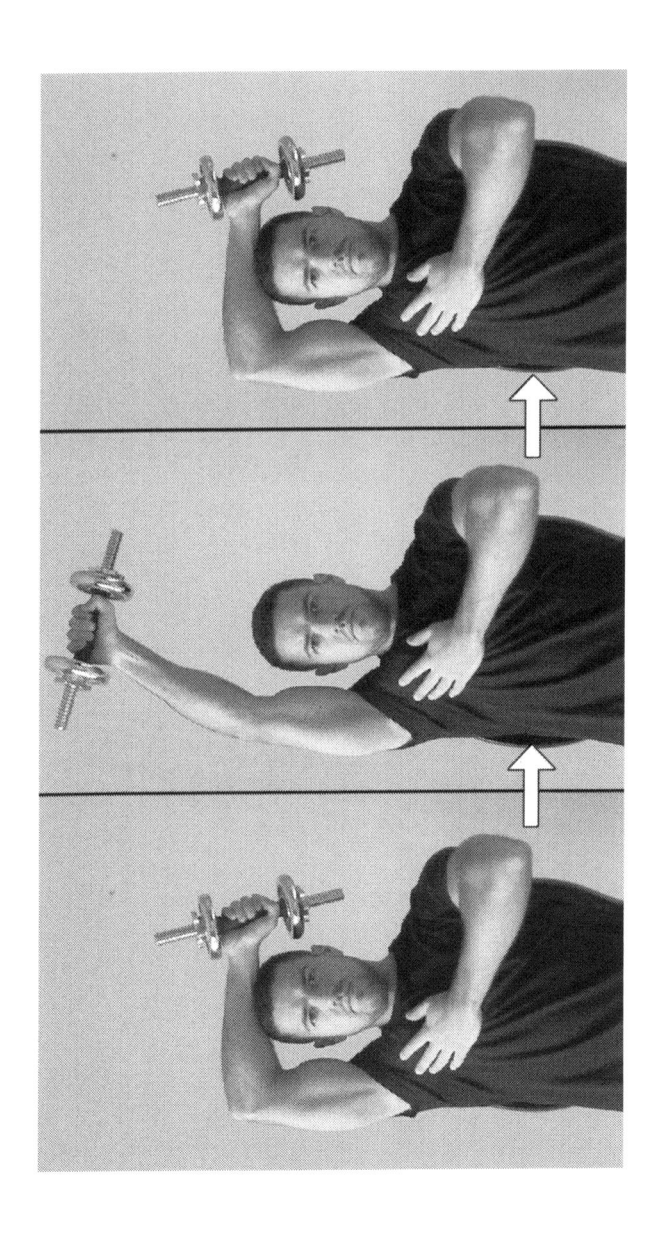

ALTERNATING ARM HAMMER CURLS   :5 SETS: 20 REPS
SUPERSET WITH
ALTERNATING ARM BICEP CURLS   :5 SETS: 8 REPS

1. Stand with your feet shoulder width apart and grip a DUMBBELL in each hand with your arms down at your side. Your palms should be facing inward towards your thighs.
2. Without moving your elbow, bend your right arm and bring the DUMBBELL towards your chest, keeping your hand and wrist in the same position so the DUMBBELL doesn't rotate at all. It should seem as though you are doing a 'skiing' motion with the DUMBBELL. This is an ALTERNATING ARM exercise so don't do anything with your left arm yet.
3. Once you have bent your right arm as much as you can and have brought the DUMBBELL up to your chest, slowly lower your right arm and return the DUMBBELL to its original position at your side. **THAT IS 1 REP.**
4. As soon as your right arm is back where it started, bend your left arm in the same manner and bring that DUMBBELL up to your chest. Keeping your elbow where it is and not rotating the DUMBBELL at all.
5. Once you have fully bent your left arm and have that DUMBBELL at your chest, slowly lower your left arm and return the DUMBBELL to its original position at your side. **THAT IS YOUR 2ND REP.**
6. As soon as your left arm is back where it started, perform another **REP** with your right arm. Continue this process until you have completed **20 REPS**. Which would work out at having performed **10 REPS** with each arm.
7. Without having a 45 second break, rotate your hands 90 degrees outwards so the bars of the DUMBBELLS are horizontally in line with each other. Your palms should be facing forwards. This is where we **SUPER SET** the ALTERNATING ARM BICEP CURLS.
8. Bend your right arm in the same controlled manner and bring the DUMBBELL to your chest; without moving your elbow or rotating the DUMBBELL as it moves.
9. Lower your right arm and return the DUMBBELL to its original position at your side. **THAT IS 1 REP.**

10. As before, bend your left arm now and bring that DUMBBELL to your chest.
11. Once you have brought that DUMBBELL fully to your chest lower it slowly back to its original position. **THAT IS YOUR 2ND REP.**
12. As soon as your left arm is back where it started, perform another **REP** with your right arm. Continue this process until your have completed **8 REPS**. Which would work out at having performed **4 REPS** with each arm.
13. Now have your 45 second break and prepare to start with the **20 REPS** of ALTERNATING ARM HAMMER CURLS again.

ALTERNATING ARM HAMMER CURLS

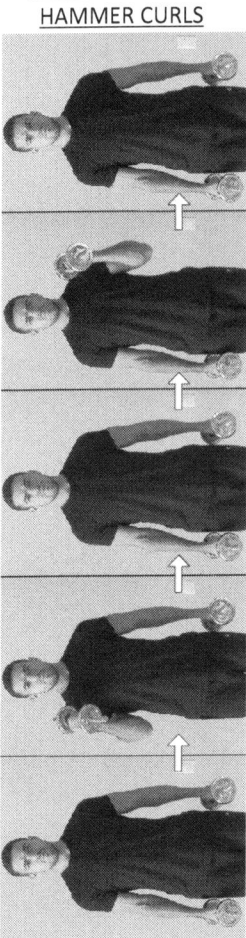

ALTERNATING ARM BICEP CURLS

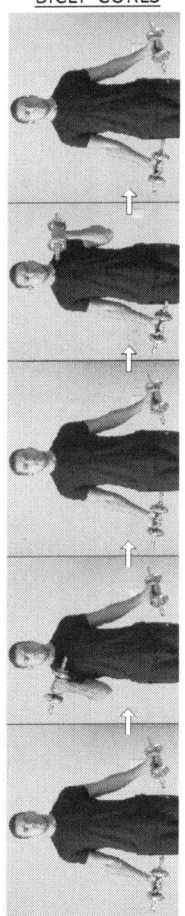

HORIZONTAL GRIP PRESS-UPS : 5 SETS in PYRAMID SET STRUCTURE: 20, 18, 16, 14 then 12 REPS

1. Place your PRESS-UP handles on the floor so they are horizontally in line with each other, they should also be in line with your chest. They should be wider apart than your shoulders. (Wide enough apart so that when you lower yourself your arms bend through a perfect 90 degree angle during the PRESS-UP movement.)
2. Grip the handles, hold your bodyweight up (your arms should have a slight bend and not be 'locked' at the elbows) and position your legs behind you. Your feet and legs should be together and your entire body (legs and back) should be completely straight. Lift your chin up slightly and look forward. This is the 'top' of the PRESS-UP and the starting position for this exercise.
3. Slowly lower your body towards the floor keeping your feet together and your legs and back straight. Lower yourself until your crotch is about to touch the floor. Your arms will bend through the 90 degree angle and your chest should be in between your PRESS-UP handles. If you have kept your body perfectly straight, your chest, chin and face won't be anywhere near touching the floor before your crotch. DON'T PUSH YOUR CROTCH FORWARD / DOWN IN AN ATTEMPT TO TOUCH THE FLOOR, **KEEP YOUR BODY STRAIGHT!**
4. Once you have reached the 'bottom' of the PRESS-UP, slowly push your body back to its starting position ready for the next **REP**. Make sure you keep your body straight and legs and feet together on your way back up.
5. Remember, the **PYRAMID SET** structure means the number of **REPS** in your **5 SETS** is **20 REPS, 18 REPS, 16 REPS, 14 REPS and then 12 REPS.**

143

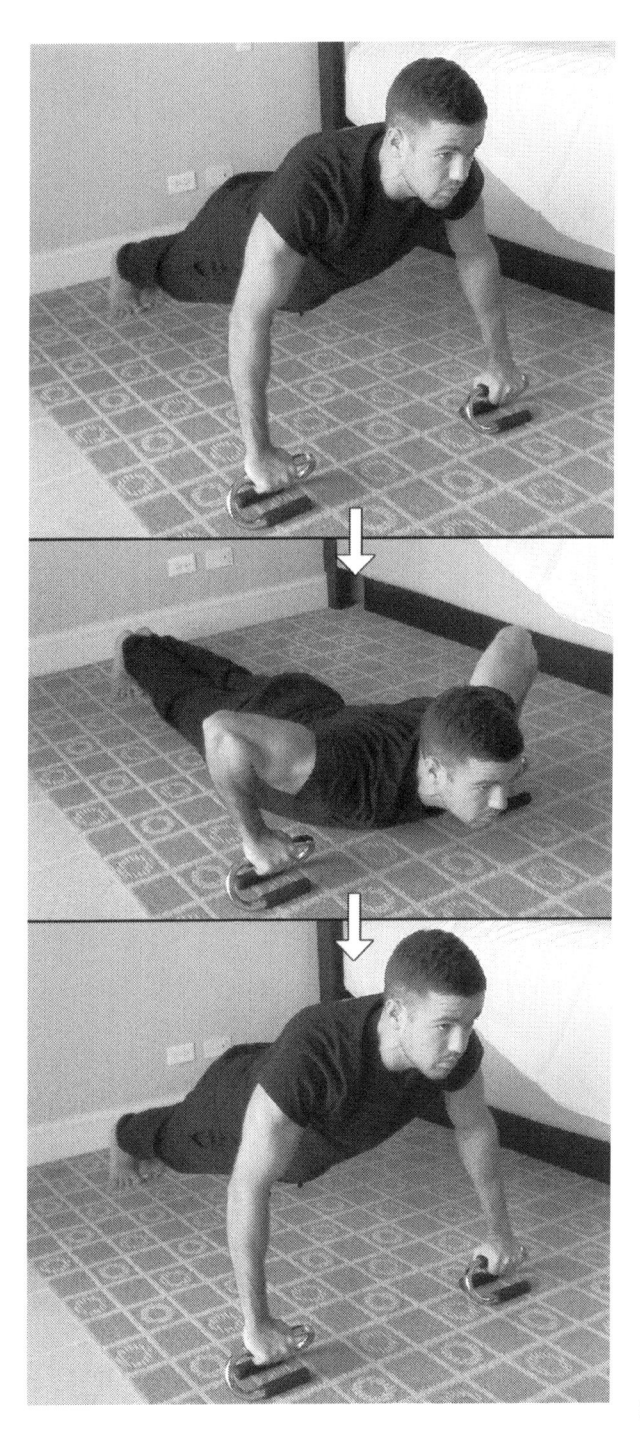

12. WHAT HAS THIS 3-MONTH JOURNEY BEEN LIKE FOR ME?

I'm writing this final chapter on March 31st, and WOW, what a 3 months. No alcohol, energy drinks or fast food, eating an incredibly clean, natural diet and working out 5-6 times a week in my charmingly cramped single bedroom. I did use a hotel gym five times over the course of the 3 months when I had to travel away; but they were mostly full of resistance machines that I feel locked my joints and restricted my movements, I much prefer my own tailored bedroom workouts. I've had no coffee, caffeine or stimulants, no sodas, diet or regular, no crisps, no chocolate, no pizzas, no chips, no ice cream, no cheese, no microwave meals... I prepared 99.9999999% of my own meals and ate more fresh, raw fruit and vegetables than I ever have before.

I didn't go on a holiday I'd half booked and paid for in advance, so lost money in an attempt to save more, which I did. By not drinking alcohol, not going on nights out and planning my meals, I saved even more money. Then during my second month I spent it all on a completely new wardrobe; which I don't consider a total failure because I have been in dire need of some new clothes. But that sudden, unexpected, late-night Internet shopping binge was a nice reminder that I am only human and despite my willpower and unwavering dedication to my strict lifestyle during these 3 months it was still possible for me to slip up if I wasn't careful. Thankfully, it didn't happen again and now at the end of the 3 months I have managed to save some more money and avoided any more impulsive shopping overloads.

Physically my body has transformed. My skin is clear, I have bigger, stronger muscles and much less excess fat all over my body, but *most importantly* I *feel* incredible. I don't sweat carrying out daily activities, my breathing has become deep and satisfying, my entire body, the joints and muscles, are all moving fluidly and freely, I feel lighter and full of life. People are saying I look much younger than I am, and I definitely don't feel as close to turning 30 as I am!

My mind and thoughts are clear and organised. Not spending every other day sick from alcohol or yo-yoing between energy drink highs and spells of self-loathing has given me time to meditate, think and reflect on *everything*. Who I am, where I'm going and what I want. I'm not governed by unpredictable emotions, tiredness or anxiety; social anxiety in particular. I haven't been living in isolation, I've been working full time and socialising; interacting with hundreds of people over the course of these 3 months. I've been in groups of people drinking alcohol, eating food I wouldn't, arguing, laughing, gossiping, judging, I've been around angry people, happy people, sad people, aggressive people, polite people and unpredictable people. Through it all I seem to have developed an absolutely overriding sense of self that renders any sort of social expectations, peer pressure or temptation utterly powerless against me. I have found it easier than ever to detach from any form of 'ego' and channel all my energy, all my passion, into *my* life, *my* pursuits and *my* wellbeing. I don't doubt that if you follow my '**BE RAD' NUTRITION** and **WORKOUT PLANS** for 3 months, you will experience something similar or even more profound.

    I've been waking up early, before my alarm on most days, ready for and looking forward to the day ahead. No, life isn't suddenly a blissful euphoria all the time. I've had disappoints, problems and felt unhappy on occasion, but I've never felt stronger, more prepared and less affected by negative changes in the world around me. Instead of turning to a bottle of whiskey, a late night and an extra large pizza, there has only been a productive response of 'What needs to be done?' and 'What can I do?' to remedy any unpleasant incidents or situations that arose. I've never felt so *in control* because I've never *been* so in control.

    I'm ready to move into the coming months with these healthier eating habits and this regular workout schedule as my default lifestyle settings, and I couldn't be happier about it. I will be allowing myself treats, alcohol and energy drinks included, but only if I genuinely *want* to have any, not because I've been pressured by life's trials and tribulations into seeking some 'temporary happiness fix'.

    To be honest, I am most excited about experimenting with healthy ingredients and actually learning to cook rather than just eating everything raw and unseasoned. I'm also interested in finding out more vegetarian alternatives, as opposed to just eggs and hummus. I know I'm going to enjoy eating a great big bacon-stuffed, cheese-coated, half-pound burger with a side of fries and peanut butter milkshake, but I can't help but know already just how bloated and sluggish such a massive portion of fatty food is going to make me feel. Firstly, it is making me address the portion size of such a meal (which even when eating out I can determine by only eating how much I want) and secondly the ingredients, what are the most natural, leanest, purest ingredients I would need to create this meal myself and to a much, *much* higher nutritional standard?

    I've had a life-changing time and wish the same for you. You have the same strength and universal energy within *you* that I have within *me*; a limitless strength with which you can claim all the self-confidence, self-respect and control you need to live a healthy life of energetic curiosity and enthusiasm.

If you have read this far I sincerely *thank you*. This might just seem like a mini fitness guide to most people, but I've been slowly piecing this book together during my 3-month journey and to me it feels more like an informative, personal journal rather than a dispassionate list of instructions to follow. I have poured myself, my honesty and my life into these pages and sent it out into the world in the hope that some good will come of it. With so much of our current reality shrouded in fear and uncertainty, at least *trying* to take control of our own lives and nurturing ourselves is the very least we can all do to improve our wellbeing, calm our souls and be at peace.

NOW PUT THAT CHOCOLATE BAR DOWN! HIT THE FLOOR AND GIVE ME AS MANY PRESS-UPS AS YOU CAN! BRUSH THE DIRT OFF YOUR HANDS AND GET READY TO GO AGAIN! THIS IS THE TIME! RIGHT NOW! THIS IS YOUR LIFE, TODAY, NOT TOMORROW, GET STARTED! GET THE JUNK OUT THE CUPBOARDS, GET THE FRUIT, VEGETABLES AND CHICKEN BREASTS IN THE FRIDGE, AND GET READY TO CHANGE YOUR LIFE!!!

! ! ! IT IS TIME FOR YOU TO 'BE RAD' ! ! !

DISCLAIMER

THE AUTHOR, B-RAD (Bradley of B-Rad TV: youtube.com/bradtelevision), HOLDS NO MEDICAL, NUTRITIONAL OR PERSONAL TRAINING QUALIFICATIONS. HE IS NOT RECOGNISED BY ANY GOVERNING BODY AS HAVING THE AUTHORITY OR CREDENTIALS TO SUGGEST DIETS OR EXERCISE PROGRAMS TO ANYONE. THIS BOOK ILLUSTRATES AND EXPLAINS THE DIET, EXERCISE AND LIFESTLYE ADOPTED BY BRADLEY OF B-RAD TV DURING A 3-MONTH TRAINING PERIOD OF HIS OWN DESIGN, UNDERTAKEN COMPLETELY AT HIS OWN RISK.

AS SUCH, ANYONE WHO FOLLOWS ALL OR ANY PART OF THIS PROGRAMME THEMSELVES WOULD BE DOING SO AT COMPLETELY THEIR OWN RISK.

BEFORE STARTING ANY NEW DIET OR EXERCISE ROUTINE YOU SHOULD ALWAYS CONSULT A MEDICAL PROFESSIONAL. TO WITNESS AND BE ADVISED ON THE CORRECT EXECUTION OF ANY PHYSICAL EXERCISES YOU SHOULD ALWAYS CONSULT A QUALIFIED PERSONAL TRAINER OR OTHER EXERCISE PROFESSIONAL.

THE AUTHOR, B-RAD (Bradley of B-Rad TV), ACCEPTS NO RESPONSIBILITY FOR ANY INJURY, AILMENT OR ILLNESS, HOWEVER SLIGHT OR SUBSTANTIAL, INCLUDING DEATH, THAT MAY OCCUR AS A RESULT OF ANYONE FOLLOWING ANY INSTRUCTION OR ADVICE PRESENTED IN *THE 'BE RAD' BEDROOM BODY BOOK*.

Printed in Great Britain
by Amazon